MW01491940

Yoga Vasistha

Vedanta Wisdom through Miniature Paintings

Yoga Vasistha

Vedanta Wisdom through Miniature Paintings

BHASKAR RAJ SAXENA

Rupa & Co

Copyright © Text & Paintings: Bhaskar Raj Saxena 2008

Published in 2008 by

Rupa & Co

7/16, Ansari Road, Daryaganj,
New Delhi 110 002

Sales Centres:

Allahabad Bangalooru Chandigarh
Chennai Hyderabad Jaipur Kathmandu
Kolkata Mumbai

All rights reserved.
No part of this publication may be reproduced,
stored in a retrieval system, or transmitted,
in any form or by any means, electronic,
mechanical, photocopying, recording or otherwise,
without the prior permission of the copyright publishers.

The author asserts the moral right to be
identified as the author of this work.

Cover and book design: PealiDezine
Typeset in 11 pts. Bodoni BK BT by PealiDezine
D4/4232, Vasant Kunj, New Delhi 110 070

Printed in India by
Nutech Photolithographers
B-240, Okhla Industrial Area, Phase-I
New Delhi-110020, India

To late Mahakavi Rai Narhari Prasad 'Narhari' who toiled
for many years to create beautiful and remarkable
paintings depicting stories of Yoga Vasistha

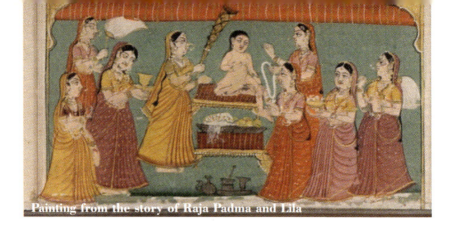

Painting from the story of Raja Padma and Lila

CONTENTS

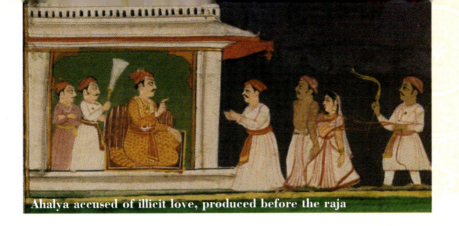

Ahalya accused of illicit love, produced before the raja

ACKNOWLEDGEMENTS

I would like to thank Ms Mallika Badrinath, creative artist, Bangalore for her valuable help in designing this volume.

My thanks to my wife, Mohini, and daughter Asha Lal without whose support I could not have completed this book.

Finally, I am grateful to my publisher, Rupa & Co, for their full cooperation and support in this endeavour.

FOREWORD

In the words of Dr B L Atray, who did his doctorate on the Philosophy of the *Yoga Vasistha*, 'The *Yoga Vasistha* is a holy Ganges of Advaita Philosophy issuing forth from the Himalayas of the Upanishads, flowing onward to the infinite ocean of the future and increasing in its depth, volume and breadth as it passes on at the Prayaga of Hindu culture, where it is enriched by the quiet Yamuna of Buddhism and the invisible yet present Saraswati of the Samakhya thought, both having their source in different oceans of the Himalayas of the Upanishads. The *Yoga Vasistha* is the sacred Triveni.'

In a lecture delivered in the USA in 1904, the great saint Swami Rama Tirtha said, 'One of the greatest books, the most wonderful ever written under the sun, the *Yoga Vasistha* which nobody on the earth can read without escaping God is consciousness.'

The cause and remedy of sufferings, self effort versus the destiny of the yogi (aspirant) to get freedom from suffering and ignorance, the teachings of Vasistha are intellectual and are meant for those who have acquired basic knowledge and intelligence. According to Swami Rama Tirtha, the remedy for all suffering springs from the mind. Life he says, as lived by the ignorant is full of misery and suffering. There is no lasting happiness as the life lived by the ignorant is full of changes such as death, deception, imperfection and ignorance. A person who wants to be happy, perfect and wise, should have a strong and ripe mind to understand and appreciate knowledge (Bramhagyana). Vasistha used a novel technique of illustrating his teachings through stories has depicted in the entire text.

This book contains miniature paintings depicting the stories of the epic *Yoga Vasistha*. The description of each story is not the full text of the original. The reader should consult any publication on *Yoga Vasistha* for full and indepth study of the epic *Yoga Vasistha*.

Bhaskar Raj Saxena
May 2008, Hyderabad

INTRODUCTION
Yoga Vasistha – A Unique Piece of Work on Indian Philosophy

Yoga Vasistha, the great epic on Vedanta is a dialogue between Rishi Vasistha and Lord Rama which takes place with the consent of King Dasaratha.

Rama returns to Ayodhya after a pilgrimage to different teerthas (sacred places) and is a changed person. He refuses to take on his royal responsibilities and spurns his worldly possessions. Raja Dasaratha is dismayed at the change in Rama. He calls his beloved son and asks, 'Why are you so despondent and indifferent to your duties?' Rama remains silent. At that moment Vishwamitra comes to Dasaratha's court. The Raja is delighted to see Vishwamitra and warmly embraces him. Vishwamitra has a favour to ask: 'Your lordship I request you to allow Rama to accompany me to the ashram. The rakshasas are obstructing the Yagna. I need Rama's help to overcome the challenge.' The Raja replies, 'I would be honoured to accompany you in the place of Rama.' Vishwamitra is furious with the Raja's response, as his heart and mind are set that the valiant Rama accompany him.

Rishi Vasistha tries to defuse the situation by asking Raja Dasaratha to concede to Rishi Vishwamitra's request. Reluctantly Raja Dasaratha commands, 'Bring Rama to the court.' A dejected Rama enters the court. Vishwamitra is surprised, 'Why Rama! Why are you so downhearted?' Rama replies, 'My Lord, I have learnt a lot from my travels. Wealth is divided unequally. While we live in luxury, many in our kingdom don't even get a square meal. Our luxury has led us to greater desires for material things. Our power has made us feel that we are invincible and that we can rule the minds and in fact the souls of the people. I prefer starvation to death!'

Vishwamitra saw the truth in what Rama said. He requested Rishi Vasistha, 'Our Rama has nearly attained self-realisation like Suka, the son of Vyasa. I implore you to teach Rama the gyaan, through stories to help him in his quest.'

The teachings of Rishi Vasistha is in short, the *Yoga Vasistha*. His teachings consist of six chapters:

- Vairagya Prakaran – Detachment (dispassion)
- Mumukshu Prakaran – Desire for attainment of Moksha
- Utpathi Prakaran – Origin of cosmos
- Stithi Prakaran – Existence
- Upsham Prakaran – Quiescence
- Nirvana Prakaran – Annihilation of the individual ego (liberation)

Vasistha says, 'Bramhan, being perfect has neither a beginning nor an end. He is the cause of the entire universe.' When Bramhan is associated with nescience it is known as jiva (individual self). The jiva is really pure intelligence and is free of nescience (ignorance).

Truth cannot be known without thinking. Thinking alone leads to the attainment of peace, liberation – 'Nirvana'. Thinking consists of logical investigation of problems such as who am I, what am I?

Yoga Vasistha illustrates that the soul is self-luminous, everlasting, and omnipresent. The next element described in detail is the mind. The mind is deceptive and egoistic with too much pride and vanity.

The third element is the corporal body formed of five physical elements or prakrati. The concept of sensation and mind has also been defined as the union of the breath of life with the body organs. If this union is merged with desire, the origin of the mind takes place.

This is why the living and sensitive plants are devoid of a mind. Therefore, it is illustrated that the end of desire is the end of the mind and leads to the end of the birth and death cycle, that is Nirvana or emancipation.

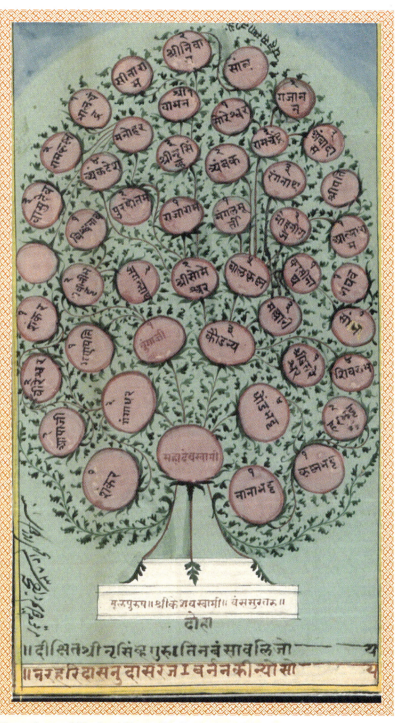

Genealogy of Narhari Prasad's Guru signed by Narhari in Hindi and Persian with date in Hijri and Samvat Era

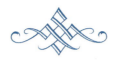

RAI NARHARI PRASAD
The Poet & Artist

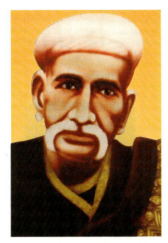

Rai Narhari Prasad
1808 - 1884

After the death of his father, Rai Swami Prasad, the responsibilities were entrusted to young Narhari Prasad. In 1820, at the age of eleven, Sikandar Jah Nizam III made Narhari Prasad, in charge of the Royal Kitchen and Mashal Khana. Narhari Prasad was found capable enough to be made commander of the Sarf-i-Khas army in 1846. During the reign of Nasir-ud-Duala, Nizam IV, Narhari Prasad organised the army in the capacity of commander. The Nizam also bestowed on him jewels. In 1858 the title of 'Rai' was conferred on him by Afzal-ud-Duala, Nizam V, on the occasion of the birthday Durbar with a mansab of 500 rupees per month.

Rai Narhari Prasad was a linguist and scholar of Hindi and Sanskrit languages. He could converse in both languages fluently. He wrote a number of books on different topics, such as *Narhari Mal*, a collection of Bhajans and *Narhari Gyan Upadesh*. But his scholarly masterpiece is *Narhari Prakash*. It is a translation of *Yoga Vasistha* into Hindi from the Sanskrit language, and it took him almost twelve years to complete the translation. *Yoga Vasistha* is a great vedantic book. The author of the book is not known but generally believed to be Valmiki, the author of the Sanskrit epic *Ramayana*. In *Yoga Vasistha*, Valmiki narrates in detail the spiritual teachings of Guru Vasistha to Lord Rama. Rai Narhari Prasad, spent several thousand rupees on the occasion of releasing this book. After critical deliberation and ascertainment by the Benaras Pandits and scholars, it was released at Benaras and distributed to the public free of cost. The book *Narhari Prakash* was widely acclaimed, by learned scholars all over India.

A learned scholar and administrator, Narhari Prasad worked in different capacities during the reign of three successive Nizams; Sikandar Jah Nizam III, Nasir-ud-Daula Nizam IV, and Afzal-ud-Daula Nizam V. He witnessed the political disturbances in the state and administrative reforms of Sir Salar Jung, the then Prime Minister of the Nizam's state.

Narhari Prasad led a happy and successful life. He not only elevated the status of the family but also established himself as a distinguished scholar. Prior to his death, in 1880, he went into seclusion for fifteen years, entrusting his entire official and non-official duties to his eldest son, Raja Girdhari Prasad.

He voluntarily retired from his duties at Royal Court and forsook his comfortable lifestyle and settled down in Devi Temple at Chanderayangutta, five miles from Hyderabad City, to achieve his lifetime goal of translating *Yoga Vasistha* from Sanskrit to Hindi Kavya (Poetry). According to my research, it is the first ever translation of *Yoga Vasistha* in Hindi. As a scholar of Hindi and Sanskrit (also Persian) he was aware that nobody had attempted to translate that great book of Vedanta to Hindi till 1856. He accomplished the task and the translation was given the title *Narhari Prakash*.

The ultimate wish of Narhari Prasad was to create awareness about the teachings of Vasistha among the general public. The *Yoga Vasistha* is voluminous and contains serious philosophy or principles of Vedanta, rather difficult for the common man to read and comprehend. Narhari Prasad, therefore, used a creative approach.

Vasistha had explained his teachings and principles through stories and upakhyans throughout the text. Narhari Prasad created miniature paintings based on the stories of Vasistha. There are about fifty-five stories in *Yoga Vasistha* and many upakhyans. (The miniature paintings, at present are available for thirty-nine stories only). Narhari Prasad selected stories having lasting appeal for the common man, who could understand and benefit from the morals of the stories depicted through the paintings. The paintings used to be on display at the Devi temple, Chanderayangutta, Hyderabad, every year on the fifth day of the Kartik month (as per Hindu Calendar) corresponding to the month of November and a function used to be held to commemorate the completion of the book. A select number of special guests as well as the general public were invited to attend the function. These functions continued to be held till 1957.

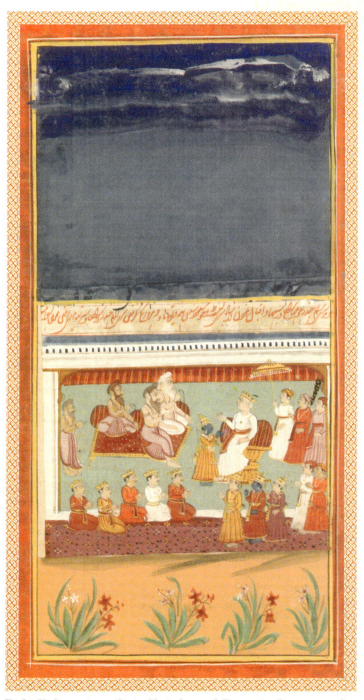

Rishi Vishwamitra, Guru Vasistha and Rama in the court of Raja Dasaratha

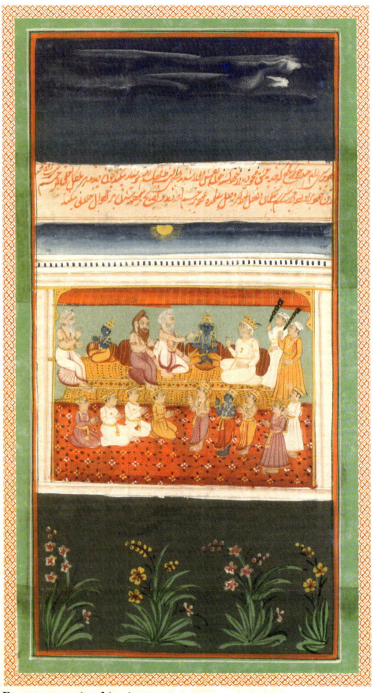

Rama presenting his views

Who is the Artist?

There is no evidence available as to who created these paintings. However, there are about twelve to fifteen paintings containing inscriptions in Persian and Hindi providing the gist and title of the paintings. The handwriting on the inscriptions is that of Narahari Prasad. The only painting – genealogy of Narhari's guru – contains the name of Narhari Prasad and also the date of the painting as per the Samvat and Hijri calendar. In the absence of the identity of the artist of these paintings, it can be presumed that the artist is none other than Narhari Prasad himself. This assumption is based on the fact that the themes of these paintings are aptly explained by the artist who was thoroughly conversant with the philosophy of Vasistha. Publishing this volume is an attempt to create awareness about the teachings of Vedanta and also to present the valuable piece of art created about 150 years ago.

Based on the Stories of Yoga Vasistha

The author of Narhari Prakash, the first Hindi translation of the Yoga Vasistha was Rai Narhari Prasad, the Army Commander of the Nizam's personal army. He had witnessed the rule of three successive Nizams – Sikandarjah (Nizam III), Nasirudullah (Nizam IV), Afzaludullah (Nizam V). He was decorated with the title of 'Rai' and awarded a mansab of Rs 500 for his meritorious services to the Nizam V.

There is no conclusive evidence that Narahari Prasad was the artist, since none of the paintings mention the name of the artist except one although the paintings were based on the Hindi version *Narhari Prakash* written in 1856. The theme of each painting is based on different principles of the Vedanta. Since Rai Narhari Prasad wrote the *Narhari Prakash* there is a strong possibility that he painted the miniatures between 1860 and 1870. The only painting with a signature is the one signed by Rai Narhari Prasad with a date also mentioned (refer to page no. xiv).

Any painting containing a message is a source of inspiration as well as a pleasure to look at. It may also sharpen one's sensibilities. A good visual with interesting details reflects life; every figure in it tells a story. To determine the real value and intricacies of a painting one needs to have the sharp eye of a goldsmith!

A survey of paintings in India by renowned specialists reveals that the art of miniature painting was at its peak when the caves of Ajanta were painted by the great artists of the second century AD.

The history of the miniature art form is very ancient and also well documented. This presentation is of the miniature paintings created in the nineteenth century in Hyderabad. After the disintegration of the Mughal Empire in the eighteenth century, the first Nizam established his dynasty in the Deccan region. He brought with him from Delhi a talented group of noblemen, a veritable spectrum of the various castes and creeds – Brahmins, Kayasthas and Rajputs. These noblemen were well-versed in literature and had a passion for art as well.

The Deccan region, comprising of the present states of Maharashtra, Andhra Pradesh and Karnataka was ruled from the fifteenth century to the seventeenth century by the Adil Shahi dynasty with capital at Bijapur, Qutab Shahi from Golconda and Nizam Shahi from Aurangabad. The various fine arts including miniature painting were growing and flourishing in those territories and came to be known as Deccan art or the Deccani School of Art. The miniature art form in each territory has its own local flavour and effect but was collectively referred to as the Deccani School of Art.

As mentioned earlier, people of many different castes and creeds from North India arrived in Hyderabad during the eighteenth century. Some of them came with the Nizam, others migrated to the South in search of a livelihood. They were exposed to the lifestyle of the Mughal court and the Rajput way of life. The Rajput culture was a part of their life. Thus they reflected a composite culture in various spheres of their life, including the fine arts. The rulers of the Nizam dynasty in Hyderabad adopted and adhered to the Mughal way of life and traditions as they were associated with the Mughal kings.

This book contains paintings based on thirty-nine stories from the famous Sanskrit classical text *Yoga Vasistha*.

These paintings were painted to convey the principles of the Advaita Vedanta, the most important aspect of Indian philosophy. Many of the paintings are impressive and elegant. In some of the paintings the essence of the visual is explained by the artist in Persian and Hindi. Although the theme of all the paintings is based on Hindu philosophy, the description in Persian suggests that the artists' main objective had been to reach out to the educated segment of the society, irrespective of their religious affiliations. During the eighteenth and nineteenth century the official language of the Nizams was Persian. Some of the noblemen were patrons of arts while others were artists themselves.

The artists of Hyderabad were in close contact with each other and also with the poets. Their paintings evolved over a period of time and have an element of all the three styles – the Rajput, Mughal and Deccan styles. However, the paintings under review predominantly reflect the influence of the Rajput style. An ancestor of Rai Narhari Prasad was also a military commander in Army of Nizam I. He had arrived in Hyderabad sometime in AD 1760 from Delhi.

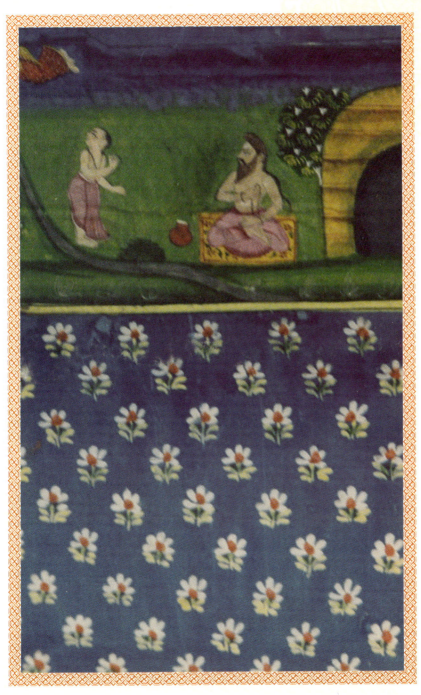

Sutikshana seeking divine knowledge; Agasti repeating *Yoga Vasistha*

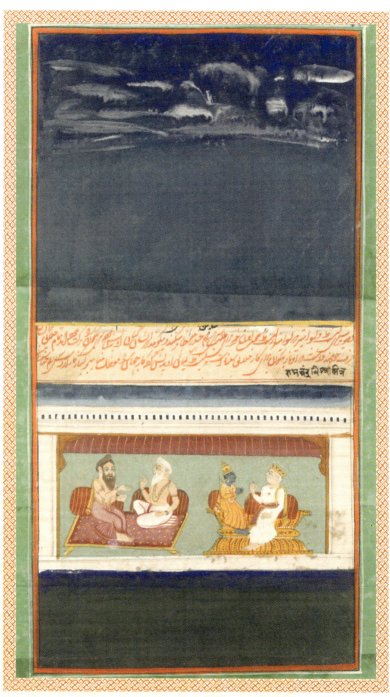

Vishwamitra suggesting Vasistha to impart divine knowledge to Rama

Hence the Deccani culture evolved due to the socio-cultural association of the noblemen belonging to the Kayasthas, Rajputs and Brahmins with the elite Muslim segment. Consequently, a fine mixture of Hindu-Muslim lifestyles and tastes evolved.

Indian fine art, in particular paintings and sculpture are rich and unique, because their contents are based on human values and mythological stories. The sacred stories and the intricate artistry make these miniatures more meaningful compared to the present day abstract paintings.

Many of the Deccan artists of the eighteenth and nineteenth century turned to personal themes from the lives of the nobles and their courtesans. Paintings depicting the worldly traits of the nobles and their courtesans, their wealth and might, was a source of income to the artists.

During the eighteenth and early nineteenth century the State of Hyderabad was politically unstable and economically bankrupt. Many years of internal conflicts between the heirs of the Nizams to seize power had led to this situation and the princely treasury was empty. As a result, the Nizams were at the mercy of the moneylenders. They also fought external wars with the Marathas and later with Tipu Sultan. Finally, with the intervention of the British who virtually took over the state administration, peace returned to Hyderabad. However, the artists continued to serve the nobles throughout the unsettled times. Other artists concentrated on religious and mythological themes based on the *Ramayana* and *Bhagvatam*. They depicted the lives of their favourite Hindu deities – Rama and Krishna.

Such pieces of art combine both the sacred and the earthliness of the gods and goddesses reflecting more creativity and magnanimity than the present forms and styles of painting.

The miniature paintings in this volume reflect this creativity and magnanimity. They are particularly unique because for the first time in Hyderabad an artist attempted to portray philosophy through art. The themes of the paintings are based on the teachings of Vedanta. The artist very boldly attempts to create an awareness of the Vedanta in his audience through a colourful presentation of the message. He deserves to be commended and recognised because he uses his art to further his spiritual cause.

One important aspect of these visuals is that the Islamic influence, if at all observed, is limited only to the costumes of the male characters.

The themes are philosophical but the artist manages to represent the philosophy very creatively through events and characters. Each character in every painting speaks effectively. The symmetry and balance of the designs of the interiors and the floor are impressive and elegant. The dominant colours used are blue, green and gold. Blue is used lavishly especially when the sky is depicted.

The characters portrayed are ornately decorated with rich attire and beautiful jewellery. Both the spiritual and worldly aspect of each scene, be it a palace or an ashram, lovemaking or war, comes through clearly through the paintings. It is evident that the artist is well-versed in depicting the royal palace of a king or the humble ashram of a saint. Nature is also depicted in fine detail especially the vegetation, animals and birds. The expressions of human behaviour reveal that the artist was a close observer of society.

Critics of the Deccan paintings are of the opinion that 'painting conceived in terms of depth does not exist in the Deccan. Although from the sixteenth century onwards, contact with other parts of the world introduced some of its spatial conventions.'

This volume will hopefully reveal the depth of the paintings to both critics and art lovers.

In conclusion, it must be noted, that the artist is highly successful in his presentation of this philosophical theme. There are a large number of miniatures throughout the country based on the *Ramayana*, the *Mahabharata* and the Puranas, but there is only one volume on the paintings based on the *Yoga Vasistha*.

Om, Salutation to the self-same reality from whom all beings proceed,
By whom they all manifest,
Upon whom they depend and in whom they become extinct.

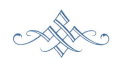

CHAPTER I
VAIRAGYA PRAKARAN
(The Divine Disinterest)

The great scripture, *Yoga Vasistha* is a dialogue between Guru Vasistha and Rama, the prince of Ayodhya – the divine disciple and seeker of knowledge. Later, the same dialogue was narrated by Aadi Kavi (poet) Valmiki, the author of the *Ramayana*, to his disciple, rishi Bharadvaja, for the benefit of all those interested in divine knowledge and self-development.

The first chapter of the Vairagya Prakaran is Rama's expression of doubts and his disinterest in life. These are narrated vividly in this chapter. The chapter begins with Rama's return to the capital after a successful pilgrimage to holy places. He undergoes a total transformation in his way of life as his attitude towards worldly life had changed. He had no desire to perform his princely duties; he refused to eat and had no inclination towards any pleasure-oriented activities. The royal servants noticed this drastic change in Rama's behaviour and informed King Dasaratha (Rama's father).

Raja Dasaratha, a loving father, could not bear to hear the report and called Rama to find out the reason for his sudden disinterest in life. Just when Rama was summoned to the court, Rishi Vishwamitra came to visit the King. Rishi Vishwamitra was one of the seven major rishis of that period. He was a friend, philosopher and guide of Rama. Rishi Vishwamitra had come to the court to take Rama with him to his ashram. Some rakshasas were preventing the rishi from performing a yagna (an important religious rite), and he wanted Rama to come and help him get rid of the menace.

Raja Dasaratha listened to Rishi Vishwamitra's appeal but politely informed him that Rama's mental attitude at that time was so disturbed that he probably could be of no use to the rishi.

Vishwamitra however talked to Rama and came to the conclusion that due to vairagya (divine disinterest towards worldly life) Rama had shunned all worldly pleasures and activities.

Vishwamitra recognised that Rama was in the same state of mind as once was Suka, the son of Vyasa. He decided to tell Rama about Suka so that he could be motivated and guided in the proper path.

Rishi Vishwamitra requested Sage Vasistha, guru of the royal family, to impart this divine knowledge (jnana) to Rama.

In this chapter the concept of vairagya (divine disinterest) in the life of the seeker of jnana (knowledge) has been discussed. The true seeker of knowledge must aspire to be free from the bondage of life, that is the cycle of death and rebirth. His vision of life should not be limited to actions needed merely for survival.

Through this well-designed chapter, education and training is imparted to the seeker of spiritual knowledge. The seeker realises that misery in life is only caused because of worldly desire, and the need for material things. The seeker is advised that anger, ahankara and ego or 'I' must be tackled and effectively controlled in order to reach his ultimate goal – liberation – nirvana.

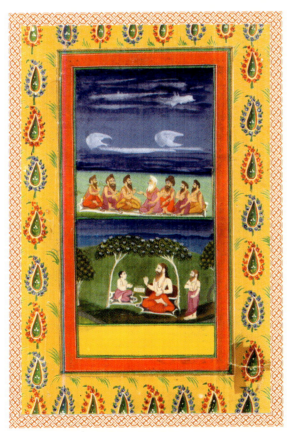

Valmiki reciting Yoga Vasistha to Bharadvaja and other disciples

The Story of the Recensions

Once upon a time a Brahmana named Sutikshan had a doubt. He approached Agasti to help resolve his problem. Agasti answered his question by narrating this ancient story:

Agnivesha saw his son ponder over the question, 'Do Vedic sacrifices or their renunciation lead one to final liberation?' Agnivesha told his son this story in answer to his question. Once a fairy named Suruci was sitting on one of the peaks of the Himalayas. She happened to see a messenger of Indra, 'Where did you come from?' she enquired. The messenger replied, 'I am returning from the hermitage of Sage Valmiki. My master had ordered me to escort King Aristanemi to someone who could help him find a way to liberation. I took him to the Sage Valmiki. The sage enlightened the king on his composition – the *Yoga Vasistha*. Vasistha had first taught this to his pupil Ramachandra. Later Valmiki recited it to Bharadvaja.'

The messenger then went on to enlighten the fairy Suruci on the teachings of the sage.

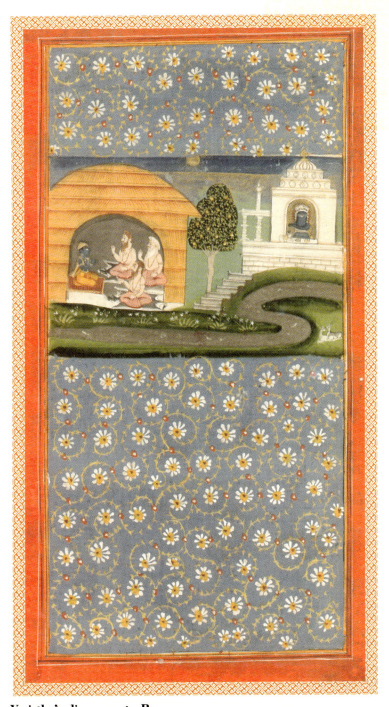

Vasistha's discourse to Rama

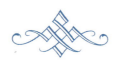

CHAPTER II
MUMUKSHA PRAKARAN
(The Divine Seeker)

In this chapter the qualities of Mumuksha or the seeker of liberation are described. Guru Vasistha explains to Rama the four fundamental traits that must be fostered by the seeker in order to get mukti or liberation.

They are:

1. Sama – the inner equilibrium of the mind.

2. Samtosa – the tranquil state achieved by the control of mind and senses.

3. Vichara – contemplation on the goal of life.

4. Sadhu-Sangha – association and living in the company of pious and saintly people.

This prakaran contains two stories to illustrate the principles that must be followed by the seekers of Mukti.

According to Vasistha the first requisite is that the mind must be trained to maintain inner equilibrium – Sama. This can be achieved by restraining the senses. Having controlled the senses and mind, the seeker reaches the state of Samtosa. The next state Vichara is attained as a result of contemplation on the objective of life. Finally, the seeker develops the traits which prepare him to commence this tough journey of divine realisation.

It is of utmost importance that the seeker puts in a concerted effort and has the confidence to reach the set goal – Mukti.

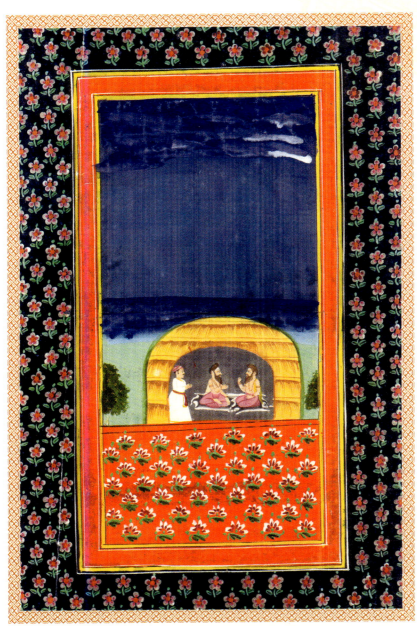

Muni Agasti teaching the art of liberation to Sutikshana

The Story of Suka

This story illustrates the character of a true yogi. Suka, the son of Vyasa asks his father, 'Father, help me to understand the truth.' Without the slightest hesitation Vyasa tells him, 'I advise you to ask the wise King Janaka the answer to your question.' Taking his father's advice, Suka goes to the city of Janaka. Janaka is informed of his arrival. Wishing to test the true credentials of his guest, Janaka makes him wait for seven days for an audience with him. On the eighth day, the king welcomes him warmly. Janaka orders his henchmen to lodge Suka in the finest room in the palace, feed him the best food and surround him with the most beautiful women to satisfy his every need. The king's henchmen follow his orders. Suka comes to the palace, but remains totally unmoved by the worldly pleasures surrounding him. He insists on knowing the truth. The king who was testing Suka then tells him, 'You are on the way to understand the truth. You have passed the test. I will be delighted to guide you.'

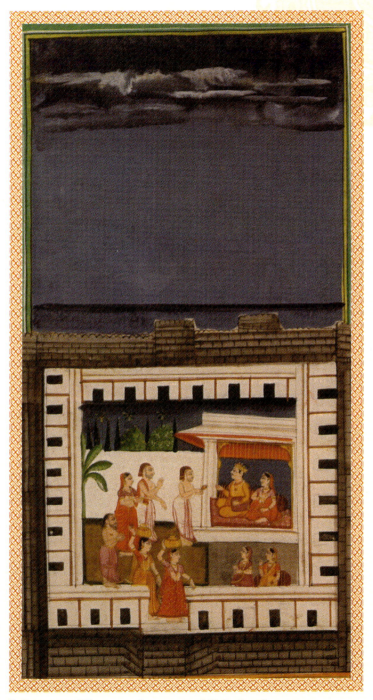

Suka, son of Vyasa at the court of Raja Janaka

THE STORY OF VASISTHA
Learning the Truth from the Creator

Bramha, after he created the world realised that there would be trouble and suffering in it due to ignorance. He therefore wished to provide some remedy for this evil. With his imagination he created Vasistha and taught him the Science of Peace and sent him to India (Bharata-Varsa) to spread gyana and create awareness among the devotees.

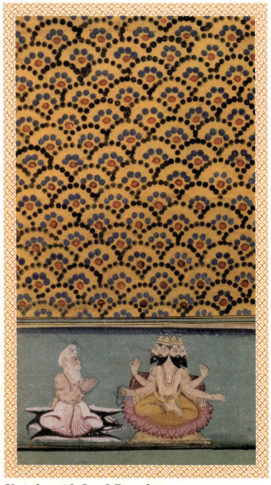

Vasistha with Lord Bramha

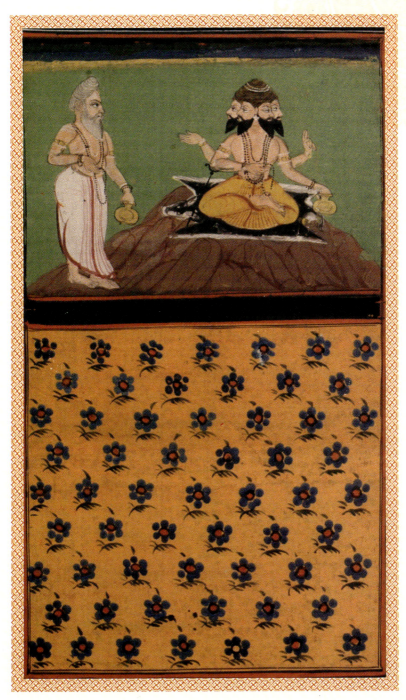

Bramha advising Vasistha to go to Bharat (India)

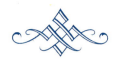

CHAPTER III
UTPATTI PRAKARAN
(The Origin)

Vasistha says that the universe exists till the perceiver exists. The origin of the universe, Sristi and knowledge is from the same source. This principle is 'I'. Dristi, Drista, Sristi and Vada are relevant as long as the perceiver exists, i.e. the 'I'.

The stories in this chapter explain the principle of 'I'. One of the most important and interesting stories in this chapter is that of Queen Lila and her husband King Padma. Through this story Vasistha has stressed that women have equal rights as men and have the same ability as men to obtain spiritual proficiency. At that time women were not encouraged to follow spiritual pursuits. Vasistha intentionally designed this story to make it clear that women should not be discriminated against in the realm of spirituality.

The problems of life have been analysed in this chapter. Vasistha advises the seeker to examine the following problems:

1. How does 'I' originate?
2. Who is responsible for 'actions' and the consequent 'reactions'?
3. How do you control the effects of actions on one's life?

The main thrust of this chapter is on the world of objects, manifestation of Samkalpa, the thought process and thoughts. The manifestation of mental activity turns into Vikalpa. This manifestation takes place at three levels:

1. Jnanakas (Absolute plane): The seeker in this plane controls mental activity.

2. Cidakasa (Psychic plane): The seeker in this plane recognises that the ego factor 'I' can be controlled only by his own efforts and steered in the right direction.

3. Bhutakasa (Elemental plane): This plane is of activities which involve desires leading to paurasa or will. Prayatna or efforts are initiated to fulfill the desires. The factor 'I' and its effect on the re-birth and death cycle is explained thoroughly. It is established beyond doubt that the ego 'I' is the sole cause for rebirth. If the seeker follows the methods suggested then he learns to effectively deal with 'I' i.e. Ahamkara. When Ahamkara is tamed, then just like a musician who practices and synchronises his voice and instrument, the seeker transforms his life into a divine symphony.

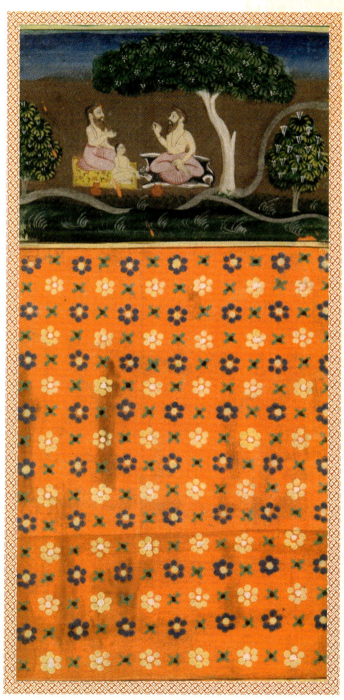

Discourse on Yoga Vasistha in progress

The Story of Akasaja

The story of Akasaja illustrates that the Brahmana is beyond the clutches of death. There was a Brahmana named Akasaja. The Lord of Death attempted to destroy him many times but was not successful. This was because he could find no karmas with which to bind him. Thus, it follows that one is destroyed only due to karmas.

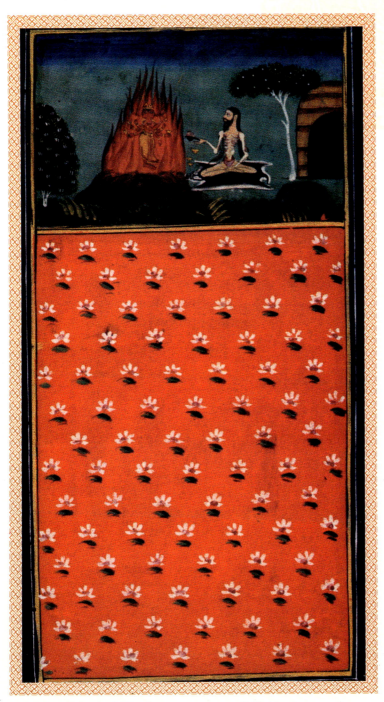

Yama, the Lord of Death, attempting to kill Aksaja

The Story of Lila

This is one of the most interesting stories of *Yoga Vasistha*. It illustrates the ideal universe, the philosophy of death and the after-death experience, the relativity of time and space, the existence of worlds within worlds, the power of desires and thoughts, and that man and woman are equally qualified to obtain supernatural powers and knowledge.

Lila was the wife of king Padma. She was so devoted to her husband that she wanted him to be immortal. She approached the priests of the court and asked, 'Is there any method by which my beloved king, Padma, can be made immortal?' In unison the priests replied, 'Impossible!'

Lila doesn't give up and prays to Saraswati. Saraswati grants her two boons, that if her husband should ever die his soul would never go out of her room. The goddess also promises to manifest herself if Lila ever needed her help again.

In the course of time, King Padma dies and Lila mourns the loss. A voice from the void tells her, 'The soul of the king is in the room where he died. Preserve his corpse.' Lila remembers the goddess who instantly appears before her. Lila implores her: 'Divine goddess, show me the experiences my lord, the king, is undergoing in the new world.' The goddess obliges and teaches her the method of seeing and visiting the various worlds, interpenetrating our world. She takes Lila to the world her husband was living in at that moment. Lila is surprised to find her husband as a sixteen-year-old king ruling over a kingdom. Her amazement increases when Saraswati speaks of Padma and Lila's previous birth.

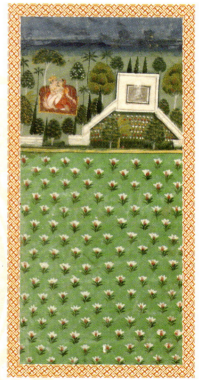

'In a small hut in a different world there lived a Brahmana named Vasistha with his wife Arundathi.

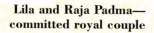

**Lila and Raja Padma—
committed royal couple**

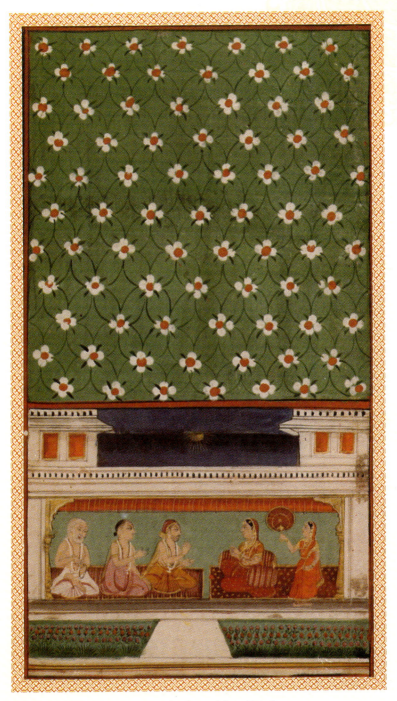

Lila consulting pundits for the long life of Padma

Arundathi had also got a similar boon to preserve the body of her husband after his death. One day the Brahmana had a dream of a king going in a procession with great pomp. The Brahmana wished that he could be that king and died. Arundathi was unable to bear the shock of separation from her husband and so she burnt herself along with the body of her husband.'

Saraswati tells her that all this happened only a week before the Brahmana pair were born as King Padma and his wife Lila. Eventually King Padma died leaving his wife Lila. Lila does not believe the story. So the goddess takes her to that world to verify the story from the son of Vasistha and Arundathi. Lila, through meditation, recollects all her previous births since her origin from the creator. Lila and Saraswati then return to the present world of the king. He is now a seventy-year-old man Viduratha with a wife, also named Lila. They manifest themselves before the king and remind him of his life as Padma. The king expresses a desire

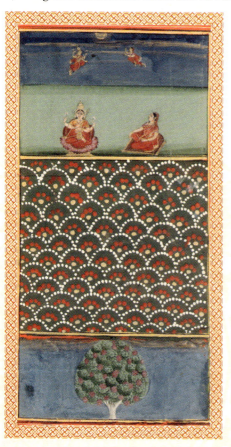

to be Padma again. His present wife prays that she be the wife of her husband, even in his future life. After a short time, there is a war in which King Viduratha is killed. His soul had never left the room in which his corpse had lain. The soul now re-enters the dead body and rises again as King Padma. King Padma finds standing before him his two wives: the first Lila of the past and the Lila of the present. The King is overjoyed and he lives happily for a long time thereafter.

Lila worshipping Goddess Sarawati to seek a boon

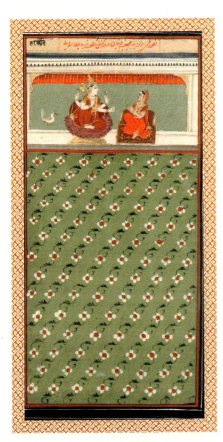

Lila imploring the goddess to know the whereabouts of Padma

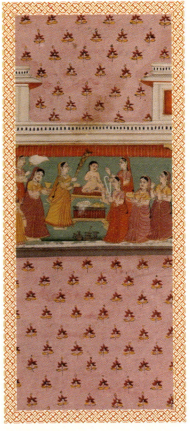

Lila finding her husband ruling as a young king

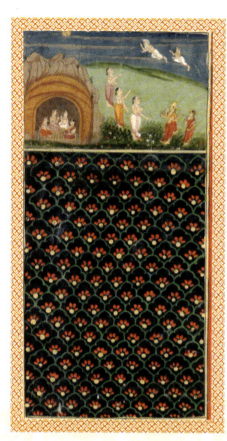

Saraswati taking Lila to various places by air

Lila mourning the demise of Padma;
Padma's preserved corpse

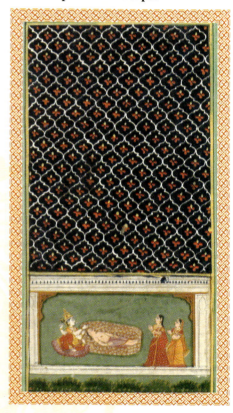

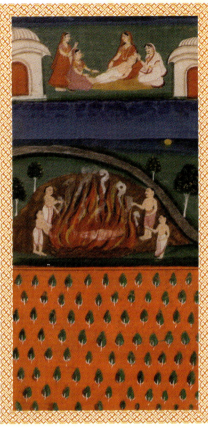

The couple Vasistha and Arundhati
too were granted a similar boon to
preserve Vasistha's body

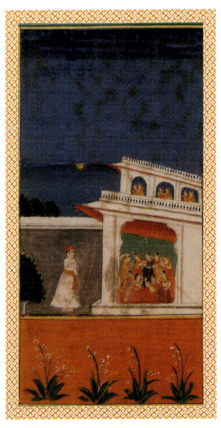

Raja Padma standing in his place
before Lila

The Story of Karkati

The story of Karkati emphasises that there is danger in this world only for the ignorant. The wise who understand the riddles of the universe and know the true nature of reality are free from all dangers.

Once there was a huge Rakshasi (demon woman) Karkati in the valleys of the Himalayas. She was a cannibal. On account of her abnormal size it was difficult for her to appease her hunger. She performed penance to overcome this. Consequently, Bramha gave her a boon; he reduced her to the size of a needle. After her size was reduced, she was called Visucika (suci-needle). Karkati regretted the penance and the reward because with her reduced size she could only enjoy one drop of blood from her prey. She again performed penance and got back her former size.

However, there was a condition to the boon; she should only prey on the ignorant. So she framed a set of questions to ask whoever she met. She once captured the Kirata king and asked him her questions; he answered her questions satisfactorily. So she decided that he was wise and set him free. The king asked her to give up her huge ugly form and take on a charming appearance. The king then let her stay in his palace and fed her with the bodies of the criminals of the state.

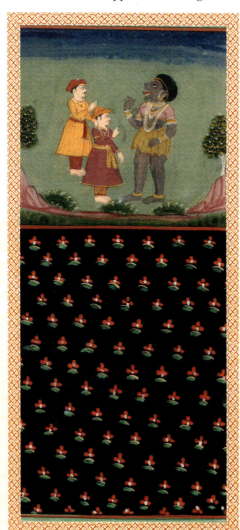

Karkati questioning Raja Kirata

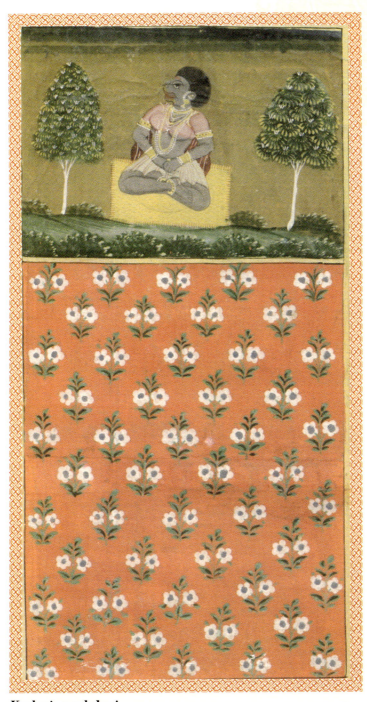

Karkati, a rakshasi

The Story of the Sons of Indu

This story illustrates the creative power of thought. Near the Kailasa hill there lived a Brahmana named Indu. When the Brahmana died his ten sons met together. A question loomed in their discussions: 'Which is the best way to commemorate our beloved father?' Their decision was unanimous. 'Each of us will become the creator of a universe.' They all sat in deep meditation and through the force of their creativity and affirmation, ten alternative world systems evolved. It was a fitting tribute to a loving father.

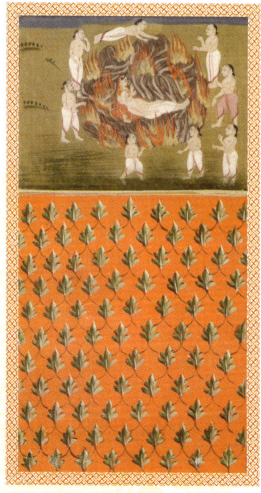

Sons of Indu

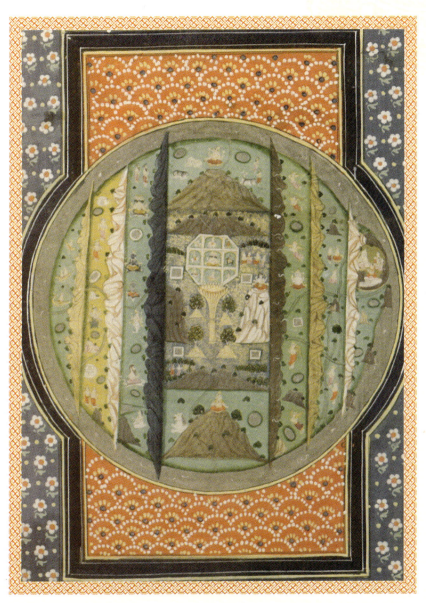

Sons of Indu evolved ten world systems

The Story of Indra and Ahalya

This story depicts how pleasure and pain depend on the determination of the mind. The body is anaesthetised from all external torture if the mind is fixed on something else. A determined mind is impervious to external coercion.

In Magadha there once lived a king named Indra. He had an exceedingly beautiful wife, Ahalya. A very handsome youth lived in the same city. Ahalya fell in love with him and he with her. He loved her very much. No sooner did the king come to know of their secret love he began to deter her from her love. Ahalya was so infatuated with her lover that she was willing to undergo all sorts of torture rather than give up her love. The lovers tolerated all the pain inflicted on them. They were so much in love that they did not feel physical pain. The king finally gave in to their love and allowed them to live together but away from his kingdom.

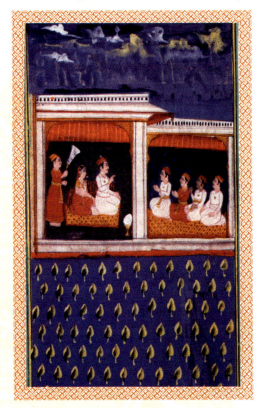

Raja Indra and Ahalya—a royal couple

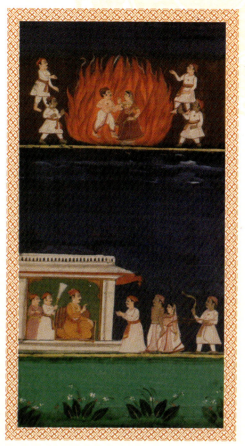

The lover thrown into the fire as
punishment but manages to survive

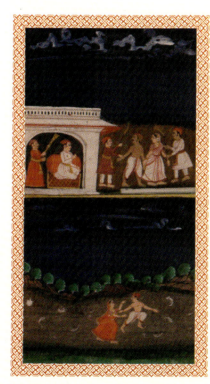

The lover leaving the city after
being banished by King Indra

The Story of Lavana

Sri Vasistha says that any seeker will ultimately realise the power of the mind. The mind is so potent that it is capable of illustrating what is ideal as well as the relativity of all things in time and space.

King Lavana lived in the Uttarapad country. A magician, Indrajit came to the court. He requested, King Lavana, 'Your highness, may 1 show you the marvels of my power?' The king granted him permission.

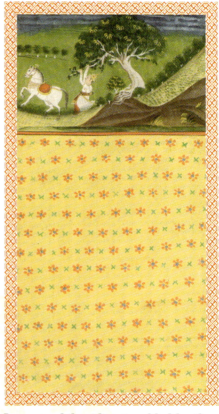

Indrajit drew out a bunch of peacock feathers with a flourish and then slowly waved it in front of the king in a mesmerising way. In a moment, the king sank into a hypnotic trance. In his hypnotic trance the king experiences a long series of events. A chief sends the king a well-bred horse. The king is troubled with the gift and wishes to get rid of the horse. He mounts, the horse and rides below the low hanging branches of a tree. The king holds on to the branches and the horse runs away. The king then wanders alone in the unknown forest. He

Lavana, while riding troubled by the horse, and hanging from the tree

gets very hungry and thirsty; at that time he spies a homely Chandala girl carrying food for her father who is working in the field. The king calls out, 'Maiden, please can you give me a portion of the food and water that you are carrying?' The girl replies, 'Sir, I will willingly give you the food and water that you ask for on one condition, you must promise to marry me.' The king agrees. She takes the king to her father. The king marries the girl with her father's consent. The king then lives in the Chandala village like a Chandala, enjoying their brotherhood but also their obscene and unsavoury way of life. The king has a number of children and lives to a ripe

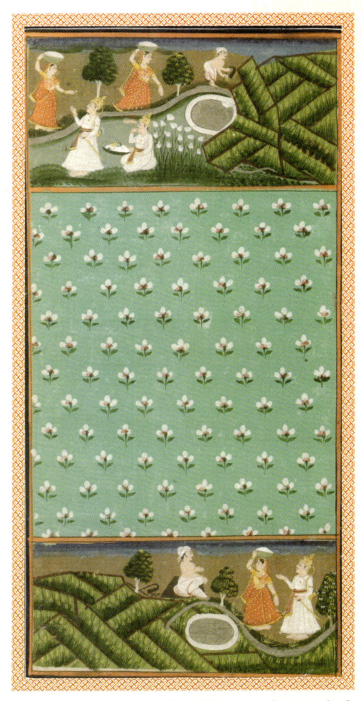

Hungry Lavana requesting Chandala maiden for some food

old age. During that time there was a terrible famine in the country. The king tried very hard, but in spite of his best efforts, he was unable to support his large family. Heartboken, he threw himself into the fire and commited suicide. He immediately woke up from his trance as King Lavana. He is amazed when he recalls what happened. Wanting to know if the experience was a trance or a reality, he visits the place in the Vindhya hills where he first met the Chandala girl.

To his utter surprise he could identify the familiar places, objects and even recognise his old parents-in-law. This was no vision; it was a reality! He was compelled to marry an ugly Chandala girl just to satisfy his unbearable hunger.

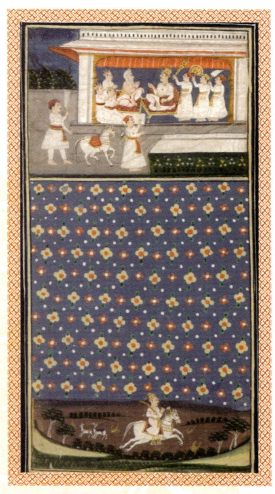

Indrajit, the magician, presenting a horse to King Lavana in his court

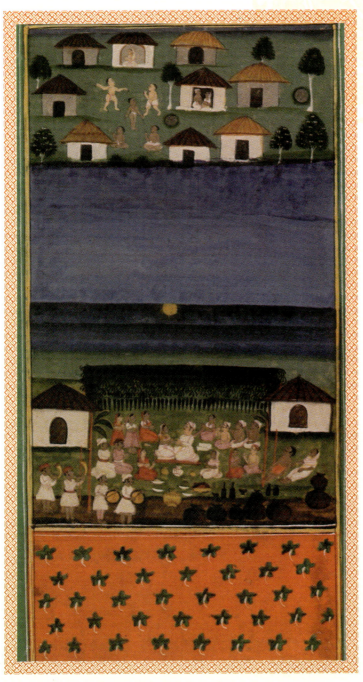

Chandala maiden giving food to Lavana on condition of marrying her; marriage of Lavana with Chandala maiden; wedding reception and feast

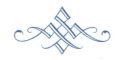

CHAPTER IV
STITHI PRAKARAN
(The Sustenance)

The fourth chapter, Stithi, deals with the factors that lead to the growth of ahamkara. A serious study of this chapter gives practical hints regarding the functioning of the ego 'I' and the 'Mind'. Through five stories the 'I' factor and its lasting effect on rebirth has been illustrated.

Guru Vasistha has outlined practical solutions to tackle the problem of ego. If a seeker follows this advice, he can overcome the limitations of life by controlling Ahamkara, 'I' or ego. 'I' is described as a great paradox; without it one is totally unconscious and yet with it most men are still unconscious and misled in life. In order to make life a divine symphony, Ahamkara must be used like a musician uses his accompanists. The musician coordinates his or her voice with the musicians playing various instruments in order to create heavenly music.

Guru Vasistha suggests that one gets engaged in Sudhama, a practice that guides one towards self-development. He also mentions that the 'I' attitude is a big hindrance during the journey to attain self-atman.

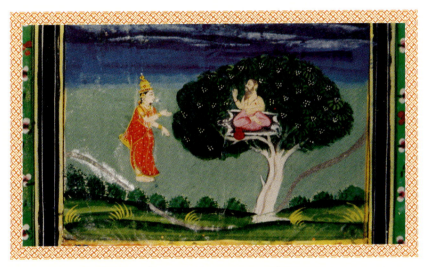

Guru Sukracharya in meditation sights a nymph

The Story of Sukracharya

This story shows that a deep desire or wish for life has amazing results. Just a mere passing wish can bring about a new birth.

The great Sage Bhrigu and his son Sukracharya were once performing penance in the mountain Mandara. During the meditation Sukra got a glimpse of a celestial nymph, and a thought creeps into his mind, 'Oh! To be with such an ethereal creature.' His subtle body leaves the physical and reaches the city of the gods. With great joy he finds his beloved and wins her love. There he lives for many years in the sweet company of his beloved. He does many good deeds but finally gets exhausted and falls down with the rain and becomes a grain of paddy. A Brahmana eats the grain and consequently a son is born as Sukra. As a boy the Brahmana is fond of deer and consequently becomes a deer in his next life. In this way he transmigrates into several bodies. Finally, he is born as the son of a tapasvin and performs penance on the banks of the Ganges.

In the meantime the original body of Sukra, which he had left a long time ago, begins to decay. His father notices the decaying body and is furious with the God of death, accusing him of letting his son die. The God of Death manifests himself in front of Bhrigu and explains what really happened. Both of them come before the meditating boy and ask him to meditate on the history of his past lives. Eventually, Sukra remembers his original form and unites with his mental body. The decaying body thus revives. Sukra turns into an enlightened soul and in due course becomes the guru of the demons.

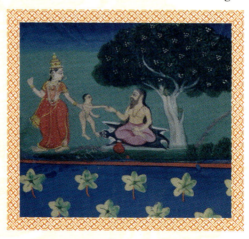

Sukracharya with Bhrigu (his son)

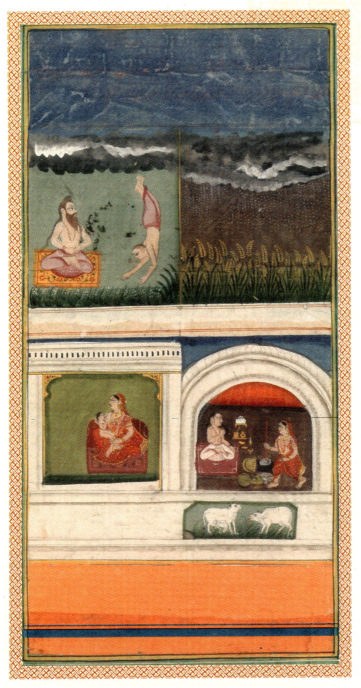

**Sukra falling down with rain; Sukra reborn as a son of a
Brahman; Sukra performing penance to attain enlightenment**

The Story of Dama, Vyala and Kata

This story explains how the will to live is the cause of all sufferings and the absence of it leads to great achievements.

There lived a wealthy and wise demon king Sambara of Patala. He attacked the gods and defeated them. The main reason for his success was his magical powers. Using his powers he created the warriors Dama, Vyala and Kata. The warriors fought selflessly without any idea of self-preservation and hence were unbeatable. The gods went to Bramha with the question, 'How, oh divine one, are Dama, Vyala and Kata unbeatable?' Bramha knowing the reason for their success advised the gods, 'Create a desire for self-preservation and desire for victory in the demons and you will overcome them.' The demons were ignorant of the true nature of self and were easily defeated in battle.

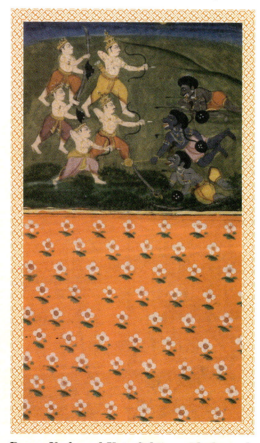

Dama, Vyala and Kata fighting with the gods

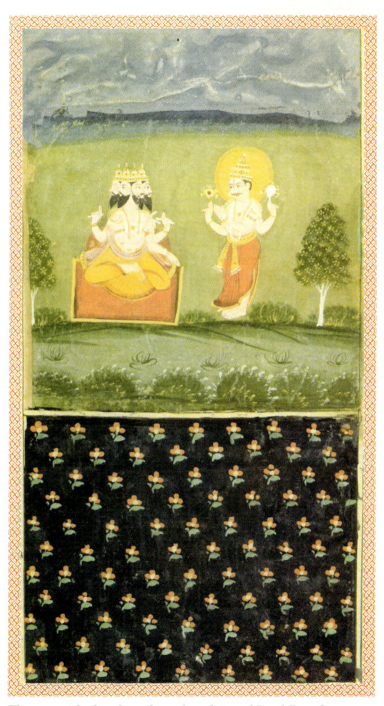

The vanquished gods seeking the advice of Lord Bramha

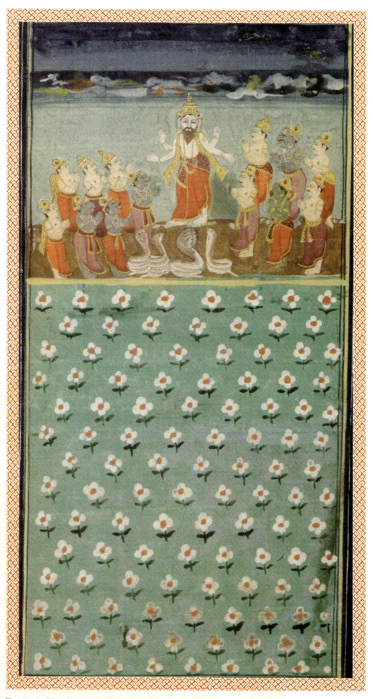

Dama, Vyala and Kata

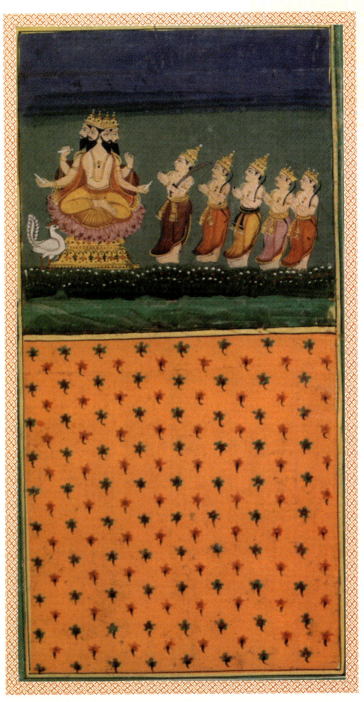

Bramha advising the gods to create a desire for self-preservation

The Story of Bhima, Bhasa and Drdha

This story is a continuation of the previous story. The desire for self-preservation cannot be created in anyone who does not know the true nature of self.

Sambara, the demon king, saw his warriors overcome by the gods. So he created another demon triad: Bhima, Bhasa and Drdha. This time around the gods were unable to create a feeling of ego in the demons because they were knowledgeable of the real nature of the self. They defeated the gods in spite of their best efforts.

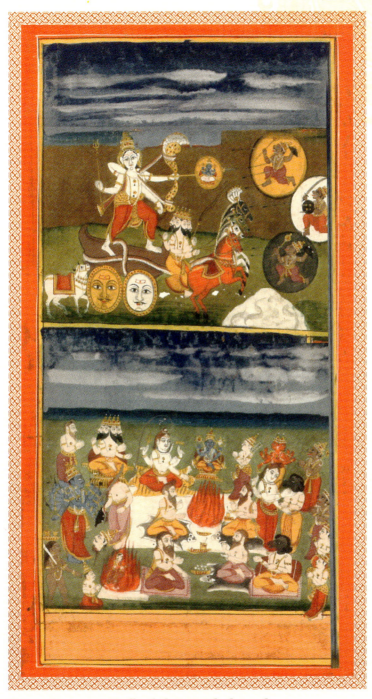

Bhim, Bhasa and Drdha fighting with the gods

The Story of Dasura

This story is designed to explain that peace cannot be achieved by undergoing penances or performing sacrifices as outlined in the Vedas. Penances and sacrifices may to some extent purify our intellect especially if performed with unselfish motives and rational thinking, meditation and knowledge of the self.

A muni named Dasura lived in Magadha. He was ignorant of the nature of the self. His father Saralman dies and Dasura weeps inconsolably. The gods of the forest advise him to search for internal peace. Dasura performs penance and difficult sacrifices but does not attain peace. Dasura then practices meditation and understands the true nature of the self; this knowledge helps him to find internal peace.

Dasura has a son with a forester woman. He teaches the boy the science of peace. Vasistha also hears one of his lectures when he passes that way.

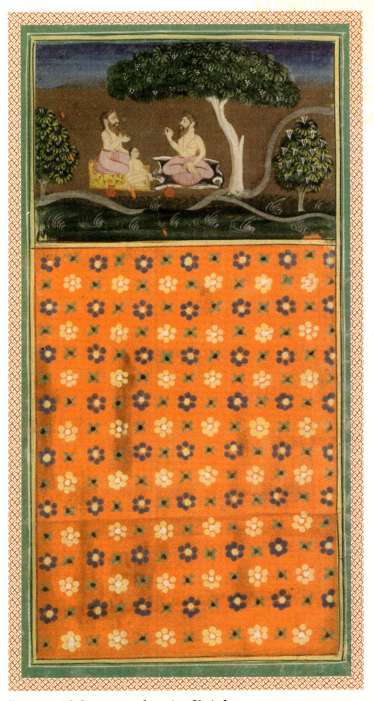

Dasura with his son, welcoming Vasistha

The Story of Kacha

This is not a story but a monologue on the immanence of God. Kacha was the son of Brihaspati. He once sat in samadhi. Waking up from his samadhi, he sang a very beautiful song on the immanence of the Brahman in everything in the universe. Later Kacha asked his father how to renounce ego: 'How shall I exist if, renounce ego, as I am the ego?' Brihaspati taught his son that ego is just an illusion and no entity. 'What is the difficulty to renounce that which is not existing?' he said.

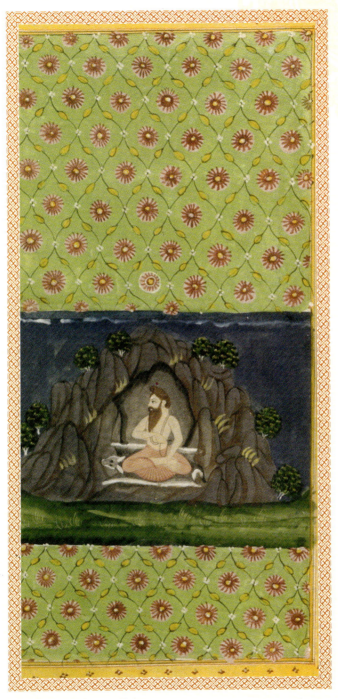

Brihaspati in Samadhi

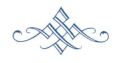

CHAPTER V
UPASAMA PRAKARAN
(The Quiescence)

In this chapter, Vasistha illustrates the techniques to control the activities of the mind, body, senses and ego, in order to reach the ultimate goal that is to quieten the mind. The main theme of this chapter is explained through ten stories.

The mind is described as a tree with two seeds called Vasanas and Prana.

The emphasis is on acquiring:

i) Jnana – knowledge – since learning helps in developing vicara;

ii) Prana – breathing – since it plays a vital role in controlling thoughts and actions.

The seeker after developing control on thoughts and actions acts as a witness, without participating in the various acts and deeds. It must be noted that the Vasanas become strong by involvement with thoughts and indulgence at the level of the body. (Jnana – the knower, Bhukta – the experience, Karta – the doer.)

The 'I' feeling and thoughts take entire credit for every act performed. Therefore, Vasistha advises and suggests various ways and means to get rid of the feeling of 'I' on the complex of mind, body and senses.

Vasistha through characters of the stories emphasises that Jnana must be acquired so that desires are tackled and controlled. Jnana is the only way by which an individual becomes strong and keeps his thoughts at bay. He also outlines indirect and direct methods of controlling the mind.

According to him Prana, breathing, speech and related activities must also be controlled because it is beneficial.

The second method suggested is that one must just become a witness – samyagaveksana – and adopt the art of non-involvement.

A person proficient in this method will not be effected by the vasanas (desires). When practised properly both the methods elevate the seeker's mental state to such an extent that the ego 'I' and its associates – the body, senses and mind – develop a stage of non-existence and the seeker realises the true self – Atman.

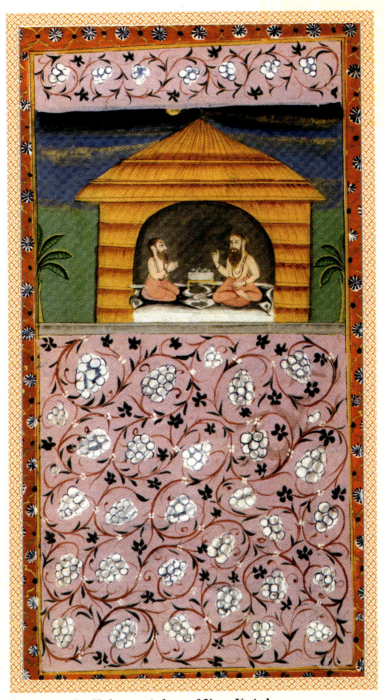

Imparting the Vedanta wisdom of Yoga Vasistha

Through the ten stories related in this chapter, Guru Vasistha explains how quiescence of mind can be achieved.

According to him the goal of human life is to achieve Nirvana. This liberation can be achieved by practising the methods prescribed. Vasistha emphasises that one should become well-versed with Jnana. Without Jnana one gets afflicted by desires and becomes a victim of his own desires. Siddhas may temporarily feel that they have reached 'nirvana' by using supernatural powers, but to a true Jnani this is of no value. The spiritual field is more important than the supernatural because then the Jnani reaches nirvana.

Guru Vasistha explains to Rama that a true seeker must have four qualities: Karuna – compassion, Maithri – friendship, Muditha – contentment, and Upeksha – disinclination. He explains that Quiescence functions at two levels: 1) Rupa – form and 2) Arupa – the formless. Rupa is powerful as it identifies with objects and the ego 'I' is responsible for all bondage and pain. Consciousness of Rupa must be destroyed because it obstructs the seeker from realising the Truth.

Arupa identifies with the mind. The entire universe including the human mind is a manifestation of Prakrati. Prakrati has three gunas – Sattwa, Rajas and Tamas. These gunas coexist and cohere to constitute unity. It is like the flame of a lamp which for its illumination requires fire, oil and a wick.

The human mind is also a synthesis of the three gunas. Of these, Sattwa is superior to Rajas and Rajas is superior to Tamas. Sattwa is pure and tranquil and has the power to illuminate; it also overcomes the other two gunas. Man who has acquired Sattwa is endowed with happiness, virtue and knowledge.

Rajas leads a person to actions; actions create attachment. This guna, Rajas, rules over Sattwa and Tamas resulting in activities to acquire wealth and fame, finally leading to suffering and misery.

The guna Tamas in a person characterises inertia, ignorance and stupidity and results in an inability to discriminate. The person lives in a dream world and with the absence of spiritual knowledge develops an evil character afflicted with grief and delusion. Hence, Tamas overcomes both Sattwa and Rajas.

Vasistha suggests that the seeker must develop and cultivate Samdrishti or uniform vision in order to transcend the duality of pleasure and pain associated with Rajas and Tamas. A person with Sattwa has an Arupa mind. Hence, the gunas represent the evolution of the mind from a psychological point of view.

Guru Vasistha says that Tamas can be overcome by practising Rajas and

Rajas can be overcome by acquiring the qualities of Sattwa. A person can also be bound by Sattwa. Hence, the final goal should be to attain Atman. Atman is free from all three gunas. Atman and Bramha are one and the same. Brahman is like a crystal clear sky which can never be overshadowed by clouds or rain.

In conclusion, Nirvana or liberation can be achieved by practising Prana and controlling the Vasanas. The Vasanas (desire) become strong by involvement at the thought level and, indulgence at the physical level. Hence for Quiescence, practising Prana and controlling Vasanas is essential.

The Story of Janaka

This story establishes that an accidental suggestion sometimes awakens the dormant discriminative tendencies of the past birth of an individual.

Janaka, the king of Videha, was once sitting in his garden. Suddenly he hears the recitation of the *Gita* by some people invisible to him. He listens closely. The recitation creates a deep impression on his mind; he meditates on the illusory nature of the world and understands the real nature of the self. He draws two important conclusions – all suffering is due to ignorance and that the true nature of self is freedom from ego. He continues to rule the kingdom but he is no longer enamoured by attractive material things. If a Jiva makes similar efforts he will be relieved of all suffering and will attain supreme bliss.

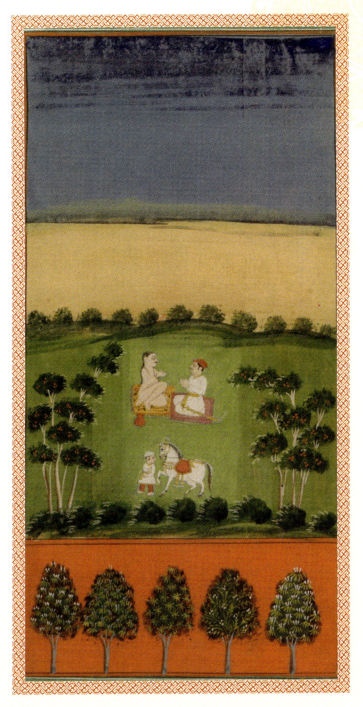

Janaka, Raja of Vaideha, listens to the recitation of the *Gita*

The Story of Punya and Pavana

This story reveals that it is absurd and futile to mourn the death of a beloved person, knowing that we have had countless memorable relations with the person in the long association of our past lives.

A sage Dirgha-tapas lived on the mountain Mahendra in the Jambu-dvipa. He had two sons – Punya and Pavana. Punya had the knowledge of truth and Pavana was on the path of discovering truth. Their father suddenly passed away. Pavana was devastated and wept bitterly at the death of their father. Punya lovingly instructed him, 'It is absurd to weep at the death of our father. You have had many lives, countless lives, as a deer, a lion, a monkey, a prince, a cow, an elephant, a bird etc. and in each life you had a father.'

He implored his brother to learn to live like sages with the sight of spiritual light, and remove false notions from his mind.

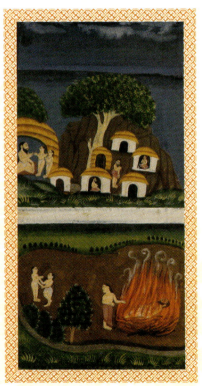

Punya and Pavana with their father; performing the last rites of their father

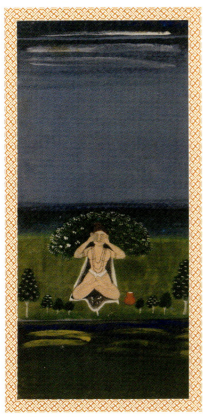

Pavana weeping

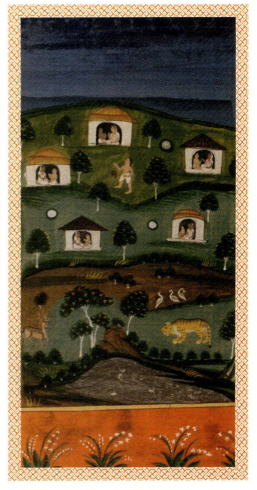

Punya describing the cycle of death and rebirth to his brother

The Story of Bali

This story illustrates how the state of Nir-vi-kalpa Samadhi can be realised through meditation and truth.

Bali, the son of Virochan of Patalok, reflects on life: 'Life is a monotonous drudgery, the same course of actions repeat themselves. Life is very unsatisfactory. My father was famous for his wisdom; he spoke of a wonderful state of existence called liberation. Liberation is the state in which one finds perpetual peace.'

Bali is eager to learn about this way of life and requests Guru Sukracharya to teach him. Guru Sukracharya says, 'Everything is consciousness. To be conscious of oneself and all that is around one is the most exciting way of life.'

Bali meditates on this truth and realises Nir-vi-kalpa Samadhi. Consequently, he becomes a truly liberated person and rules wisely over his kingdom. Then Lord Vishnu appears and confers his blessings upon him.

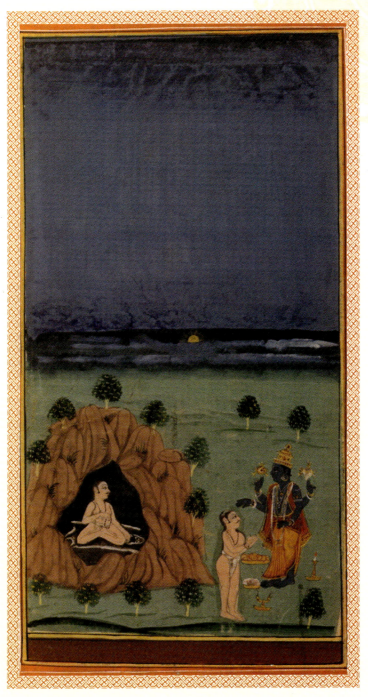

**Bali meditating in the state of Nir-Vi-Kalpa Samadhi;
Lord Vishnu conferring his blessings on Bali**

The Story of Prahlada

This story illustrates that man can realise the self only by applying himself and through meditation. The grace of God or that of a teacher cannot confer the knowledge of self to a person. A person must endeavour to achieve this on his own.

Once Vishnu defeated some demons and killed their Lord, Hiranya-kasipu. Prahlada, the son of the killed demon, was impressed and became a devotee of Sri Vishnu. Vishnu, pleased with his devotion, appeared before him and said, 'Prahlada, choose a boon as a reward for your devotion.' Prahlada thought deeply and said, 'My Lord I wish to realise the true nature of self.' Vishnu answered, 'You will be able to realise the self only by your own effort and meditation. No God or teacher can confer this knowledge on you.'

Prahlada meditates and attains a state of Samadhi. The bliss of Samadhi makes him forget his royal duties. Meanwhile, anarchy prevails in his kingdom due to his neglect. Vishnu wakes him up from his Samadhi and orders him, 'Your duty is to rule over your kingdom as an ideal and wise ruler.' Prahlada immediately recognises his true duty and carries out Lord Vishnu's orders.

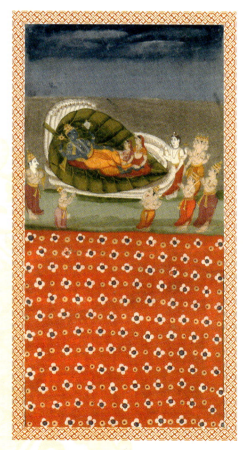

Gods requesting Lord Vishnu to protect Prahlada

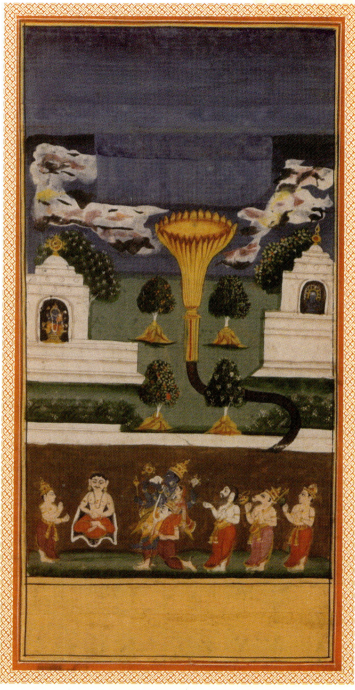

**Lord Vishnu descending to Patal-Loka; Prahlada awakened by
Lord Vishnu to perform his duties**

The Story of Gadi

This is an interesting story that illustrates the creative power of Maya. Maya creates a real historical event experienced by an individual mind, a few moments before its actual occurrence.

A Brahmana named Gadi was very keen to know the nature of Maya. The Brahmana regularly worshipped Vishnu. Vishnu granted him a boon – the knowledge of the nature of Maya.

One day while he was bathing, he dipped his head in the river and sees a vision that he is ill at home and then he dies. He is born again as an ugly, black son of a Chandala woman. After sometime he marries a Chandala and has several children.

Once, he passes through a place known as 'Kira'. He is picked up by an elephant, which has been left loose to elect a king, in the place of the king who was dead. After the elephant picks him up he is inducted as the new king. He rules over the kingdom for sometime, before it is discovered, that he is a Chandala by birth. The higher caste subjects walk into fire to perform Prayascihta, because a Chandala king ruled them. The king is sorrowful on seeing this horrific scene and jumps into the fire. The intense pain awakens him and he is again Gadi bathing near the river. The whole event occurred within a few seconds of his dipping his head in the water.

After a few months he meets a traveller who narrates the story of the Chandala king, which occurred during his travels. The coincidence was astounding. Gadi verifies that it actually happened in the physical world. Such is the amazing power of Maya!

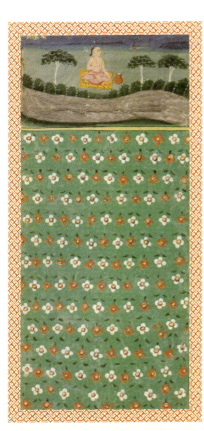

Gadi keen to know about Maya

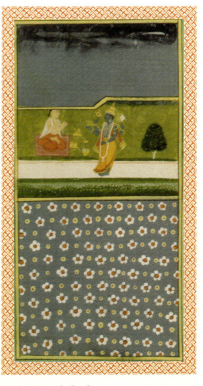

Vishnu and Gadi

The Story of Uddalaka

This story teaches how the mind of a person who has reached self-realisation, can be controlled by meditation and by the practise of the control of the vital prana (vital air).

A muni named Uddalaka decides to experience the state of Samadhi. He realises that the mind is a great impediment in his experience because the mind is forever straying. This prevents him from discovering the nature of the self. He practises the control of the mind by meditation and by the control of prana, and realises the state of Samadhi known as Sattawa Samanya or pure consciousness.

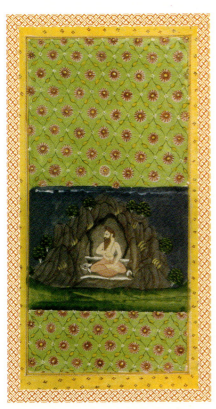

Uddalaka Muni in meditation

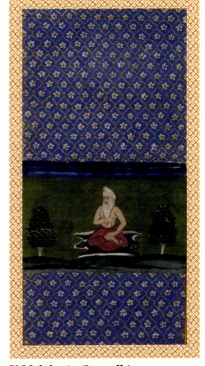

Uddalaka in Samadhi

The Story of Suraghu

This story illustrates how tranquility can be achieved even while performing routine duties. The muni Mandavya pays a visit to King Suraghu of Kirta. The king requests him to teach him how to experience serenity in the middle of the hustle and bustle of worldly affairs. The muni teaches him that the self is the reality which persists after every object is eliminated. Suraghu starts experimenting with the teaching and succeeds in attaining calmness of mind.

Once, he receives a king Parigha, and teaches him how to enjoy the state of Samadhi even while busy performing his worldly duties. King Parigha realises the self and Ananda. All his desires are annihilated and he attains supreme bliss.

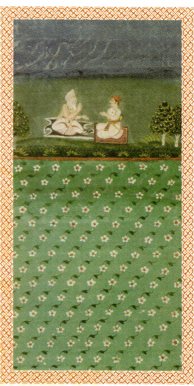

Raja Suraghu imploring Muni Mandavaya

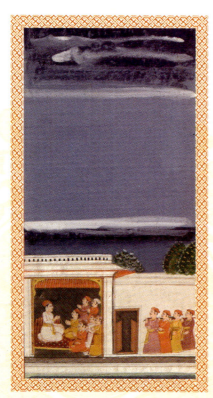

Raja Suraghu welcoming Raja Parigha and instructing him

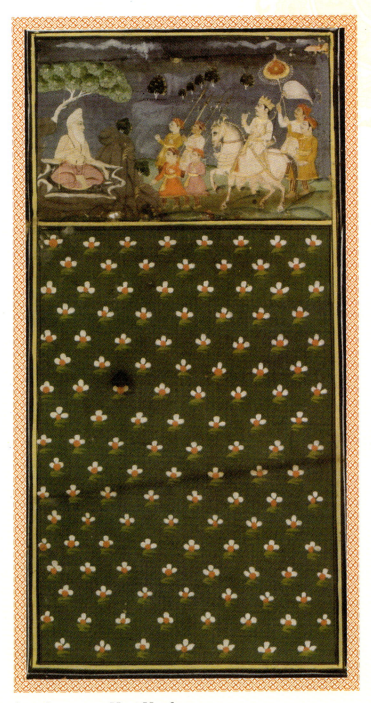

Suraghu goes to Muni Mandavya

The Story of Bhasa and Vilasa

This story teaches that one cannot be at peace unless the mind is under control and only then can the self be realised.

A great rishi, Atri lives with his pious wife Anasuya on the Sahya mountain. They have two sons – Bhasa and Vilasa. After the death of their parents, Bhasa and Vilasa go in two different directions to perform penance. After sometime the brothers meet. Vilasa asks Bhasa, 'How have you been doing, brother? Did you find peace?' To which Bhasa replies, 'A Jiva does not get enough peace in the world until he has lost his ego. He then attains Atmaveda.'

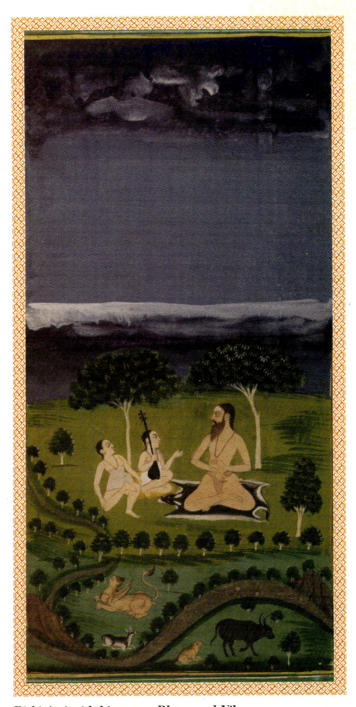

Rishi Atri with his sons—Bhasa and Vilasa

The Story of Muni Vitahavya

This story narrates how to attain self-realisation, the best state of existence. Vitahavya was a muni in the Vindhya hills. Vitahavya performed many rites prescribed by the sastras but he could not attain peace. He decides in his quest for peace that he has to realise the state of Nir-vi-kalpa Samadhi. He reaches the state of Samadhi by addressing his mind and senses and controlling them; he remains in the state of Samadhi for a very long time. During the time of his Samadhi his body is covered by earth. When he wakes up from his Samadhi he is unable to walk. He remains unperturbed and creates another world through the power of thought. He lives in the newly created world as a liberated man. Ultimately, he realises that the highest state of existence is Atma. Atma is always illuminating, pure and it is the true nature of Ananda.

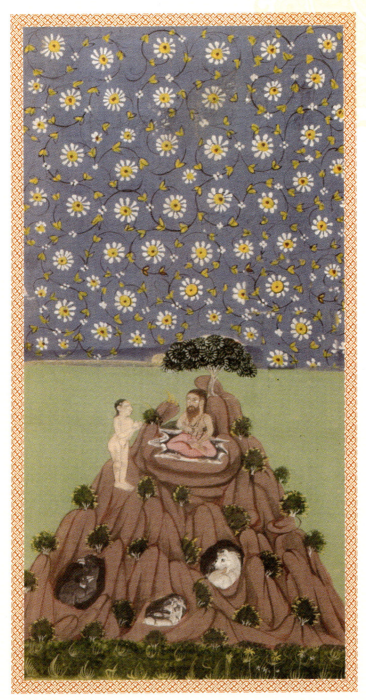

Muni Vitahavya in the state of Nir-Vi-Kalpa Samadhi

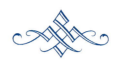

CHAPTER VI
NIRVANA PRAKARAN
(The Final Liberation)

In this chapter Guru Vasistha elucidates on his deepest thoughts on Nirvana through fifteen convincing stories using language with style and flair.

Time and space both change, but are relative to one another through one unchanging principle or entity. This is because the cosmos is in a state of dynamic equilibrium.

Guru Vasistha made a significant observation that there is nothing like time and space. The absolute Bramhan is existence – an existence where knowledge and bliss are merged with the very existence itself. Bramhan is non-dual, transcends all and is immutable. Bramhan is changeless and has no beginning and no end.

The important topics discussed in this chapter are:

1. Prana Vidya – the science of breathing
2. Guru Sisya relationship – the guru guides the sisya
3. True renunciation
4. Purity of mind
5. The seven stages the seeker must pass through to reach the goal of nirvana.

Nirvana – the ultimate goal of life – can only be achieved by restraining worldly desires and controlling the self from indulging in worldly pleasures. The 'I' feeling is associated with all manifestations. The illusions of citta (mind) creates a desire for worldly objects. The desire continues as long as the 'I' and 'mine' feeling exists.

The seeker, however, engaged in meditation encounters no such desires and longing for pleasure. There is no duplicity of mind in the seeker as he is meditating on the all-pervading Atman – the infinite Bramhan. A seeker, makes no distinction between friend and enemy.

In this chapter Guru Vasistha illustrates the approach of a Jnani or seeker in his journey towards his ultimate goal 'Nirvana'.

The way in which the topic is presented is one of the masterpieces of this great scripture. It outlines how a seeker may wander aimlessly unless he or she has an able guru to provide proper guidance. It also emphasises that the Jnani must renew his or her knowledge periodically to avoid

Avidya or wrong notions. Avidya leads to acts of deceit, anger, greed and Ahamkara. To reach the goal one has to overcome all these acts.

On Rama's request, Guru Vasistha explains the two paths leading to elimination of Vasanas and desires. The two techniques are Jnana and Prana. Vasistha substantiates that Yoga is the best technique to control the mind and to completely cross over the ocean of Samskara. Vasistha says that Yoga is not the control of only Prana and explains the other aspects of Yoga in this chapter.

Nirvana Prakaran is divided into two parts. This prakaran is intelligently and artistically designed; apt phrases and verses are used.

The most fascinating story in the entire text is the story of Rani Chudala and Raja Sikhadhvaja. The importance of this story is that it clearly establishes that a woman is equal to a man in every walk of life. This story is significant even today because it invalidates the concept that in ancient India women were discriminated against. Chudala was not only spiritually superior to her husband, but she also ruled the country in the absence of Raja Sikhadhvaja.

The Story of Kag-Bhusunda

Kag-Bhusunda in the puranic explanation is a crow. In reality, this is not the case; Kag-Bhusunda is the name of a person, an individual denoted as man of the *Yoga Vasistha*.

This story explains how the efficiency and proficiency of Prana and Kundalini is likely to lead to an infinitely long and healthy life.

Once Vasistha in the assembly of gods comes to know of Kag-Bhusunda who is said to be enjoying a very long life, longer than any other person. Vasistha is inquisitive to meet this person and learn his secret, so he goes to Kailasa where Kag-Bhusunda was said to reside under the Kalpa tree. Kag-Bhusunda welcomes him. Vasistha is eager to learn how he survives universal destruction. Kag-Bhusunda then narrates the story of his birth, the wonderful experiences he had and how he had witnessed a number of births and rebirths of Vasistha, Vishnu, Buddha, Rama and Krishna in his life-time. He concludes: 'I believe with firm faith, that I am a non-doer (Akarta), hence, I am bound to nothing and am truly liberated.'

Classification regarding Kag-Bhusunda: It is generally considered in Indian mythology that Kag-Bhusunda was a crow, but the author of *Yoga-Vasistha*, did not mention him as a crow.

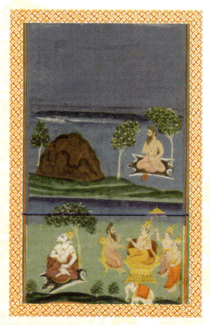

**Vasistha learning about Bhusunda
in the company of gods**

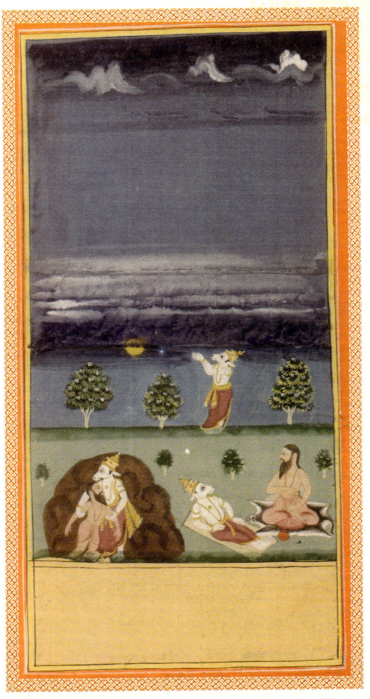

Bhusunda welcoming Vasistha; Bhusunda narrating his life history; Bhusunda as a liberated person

The Story of Deva-Puja (Worship of God)

That the best form of worship is one in which there is no external show, is touched upon in this story.

Once Vasistha goes to Kailasa and worships Shiva. Shiva is pleased with the sincerity of his worship and appears with his wife Parvati, before him. Vasistha feels truly blessed and asks, 'My lord, what is the best form of worship?' Shiva replies, 'The worship of self is the best form of worship and the knowledge of self is the best form of worshipping the self.'

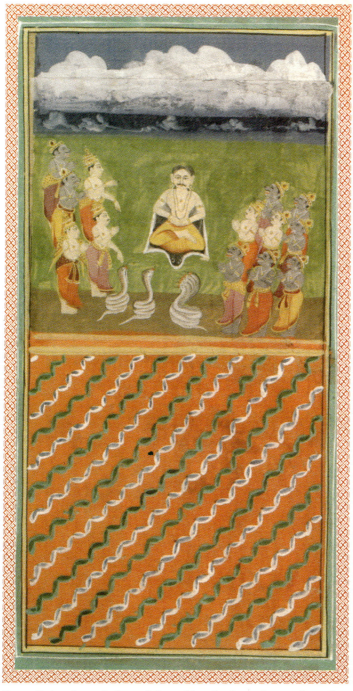

Deva-Puja—knowledge of the self is the best form of worship

The Story of Arjuna

This story predicts that in future the world will be ruled by evil-doers but Vishnu would come in the form of Krishna and kill them. Arjuna in the battlefield of *Mahabharata* would hesitate to kill. Krishna would teach him the right attitude towards life. Krishna would teach him how to destroy attachment and remain in the true state of self. Arjuna would acquire this knowledge and do his duty, as prescribed by Dharma.

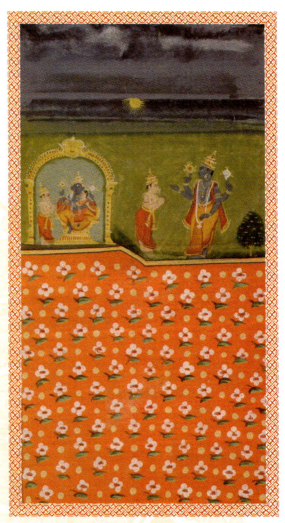

Arjuna and Lord Krishna as Vishnu

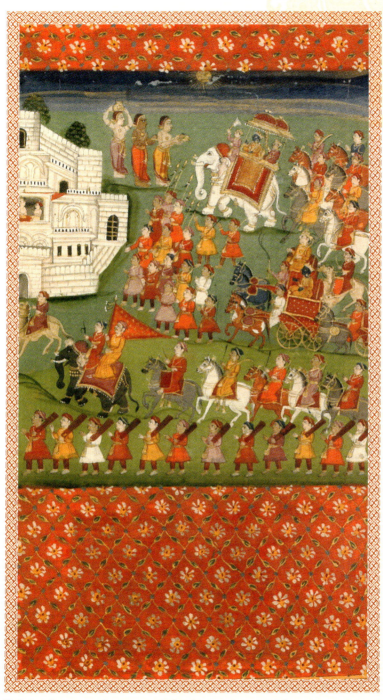

Vishnu directing Arjuna to fight for protecting Dharma

The Story of Bhagiratha

This story shows how a truly liberated person has the strength of character and the traits to perform all day-to-day worldly activities for the good of others in spite of being detached from the world.

Bhagiratha is the great king who brought the Ganga down to the earth. At the time, Bhagiratha realises the unreality of worldly possessions and goes to Guru Tritula to learn about detachment and the knowledge of self. When he attains the knowledge of self he gives away his entire kingdom and property in charity and goes to a secluded place to meditate. There he realises the ultimate truth and lives in bliss and peace.

Once he passes through the country he had ruled earlier. The ruling king had just died and the people were about to choose another ruler. The people recognise Bhagiratha and request him to be their king once again. Bhagiratha concedes to their request in order to provide them with a just and wise ruler.

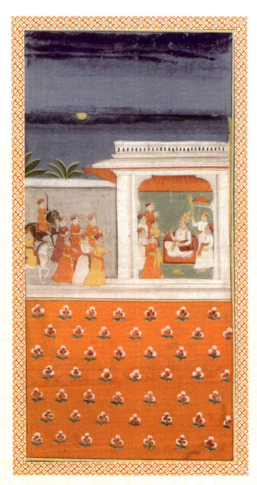

Raja Bhagiratha, a great king, conducting his court

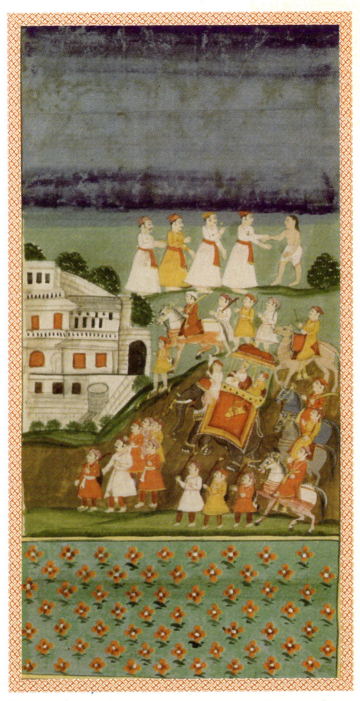

Bhagiratha renounces the world but his people again elect
him as their ruler

The Story of Chudala and Sikhadhvaja

This is one of the most interesting and fascinating stories of the *Yoga Vasistha*. It is fascinating and educative as it concerns women. This story clearly shows that a woman is not excluded from the temple of wisdom. A woman has an equal right to knowledge of the self. In fact if she makes an effort, not only can she realise the self, but can also put her husband on the right path. Renunciation of external worldly things and deeds do not result in self-realisation. It is the renunciation of internal desire and a craving for it that causes it. Queen Chudala is an ideal ruler, but she is above the turmoil of life. She is at peace within, a shining example of a truly liberated individual. This is her story.

The King of Malava, Sikhadhvaja, was married to Chudala the princes of Saurashtra. After a happy life, full of love and enjoyment, they both become dissatisfied with worldly pleasures and decide to seek knowledge of self. Chudala is more enthusiastic and discriminative and succeeds in getting the true vision of life. Her face glows with a lustre due to her inner contentment and peace. However, the king is unable to realise the self and is unable to tolerate her joyousness. Chudala tries to help him, but he doesn't give any importance to her ideas. She then tries to use her supernatural powers, but still fails to make him peaceful from within.

The king then performs different religious ceremonies, but they don't give him any solace. He then renounces his kingdom and all worldly things and retires to the forest. His wife asks him not to go but he does not pay attention to her entreaty. In the forest he puts himself through severe austerities.

In the meantime, Chudala rules over the kingdom well and wisely. Filled with compassion for her husband, she visits him secretly; she intends to teach him the way of self-realisation. She knows that he will not take her seriously, so using her yogic powers she transforms herself into a saintly person called Kumbha. The king accepts Kumbha as his teacher and learns the secret of self-realisation from him. He learns that the way to self-realisation is not by the renunciation of external things but by the renunciation of desires. Desire is the root of all evil. He treats Kumbha as his Guru.

Now and then the queen leaves the king and returns to her kingdom to attend to her royal duties. The king having learnt the true nature of self, experiences Samadhi and is liberated from all feelings. The queen as Kumbha tests him in many ways. One day she tells the king, 'I am cursed by Durvasa to be a woman at night and a man by day. I'm extremely

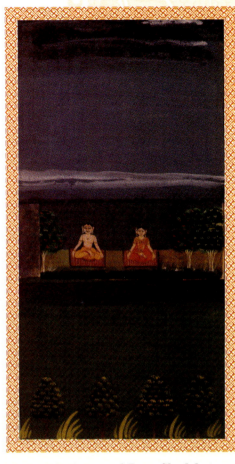

King Sikhadvaja and Rani Chudala in

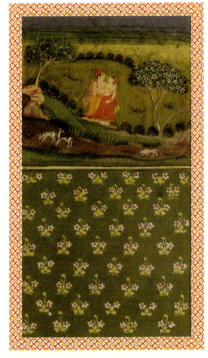

Raja Sikhadvaja and Rani Chudala—an ideal royal couple

unhappy.' The king replies, 'You must not be upset by this change; what cannot be cured must be endured.'

At night Kumbha changes into Mandanika. She tells the king, 'It is natural for a young woman to have a husband. Will you marry me?' The king sees neither loss nor gain in this move, and marries her. They pass the nights in conjugal bliss. To test the king's detachment, Mandanika with her yogic powers, conjures a lover. She throws herself into her lover's arm and arranges that the king sees her in a compromising situation. The scene doesn't perturb the king in any way. He keeps a balanced mind and does not fly off in a rage.

With this and other such challenges, Chudala trains Sikhadhvaja in the art of living. Eventually, he becomes a perfectly free and wise man and returns to rule the kingdom he had renounced.

Sikhadhvaja means one with peacock flag. According to Hindu belief, Manas is bestowed with peacock colour.

Chudala means resting on head. The pineal gland is located in the neck near the head and controls Budhi (Intelligence).

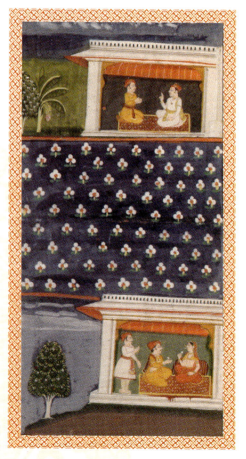

Raja Sikhadvaja and Rani Chudala ruling the kingdom

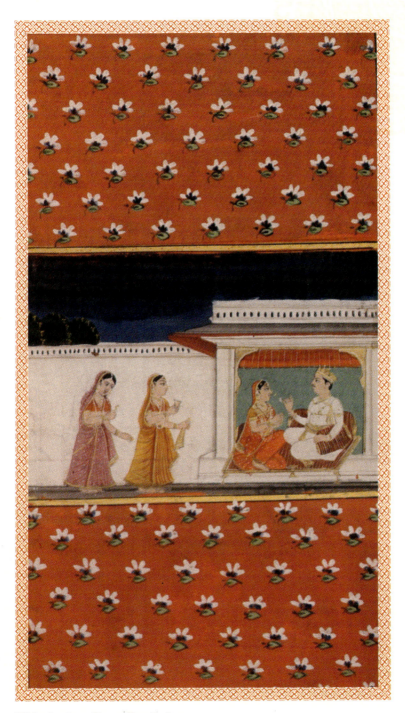

Sikhadvaja ruling effectively

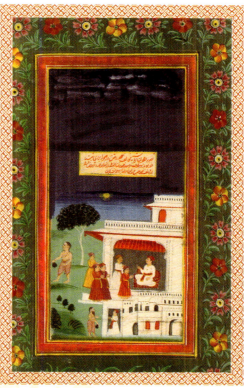

Sikhadvaja decides to renounce his kingdom

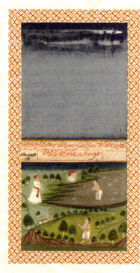

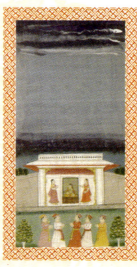

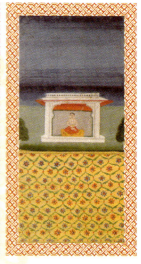

Raja Sikhadvaja renouncing his royal robes in the forest

Chudala takes over the reins of the kingdom

Chudala with her yogic powers tracking Sikhadvaja

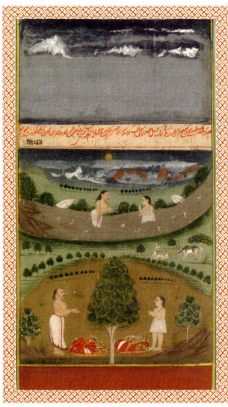

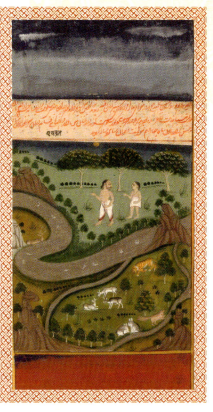

Chudala arriving as Kumbha; Raja doing Namaskar to Kumbha

After explaining about renunciation, Kumbha bidding farewell with a promise to return

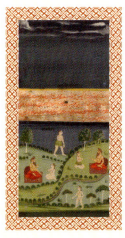

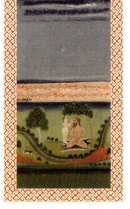

Chudala as Kumbha describing past history; Kumbha blessing Sikhadhvaja

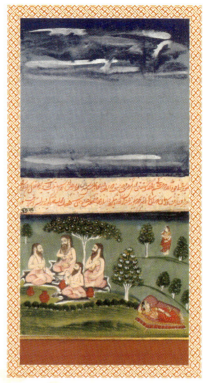

Kumbha's meeting with Rishi Durvasa

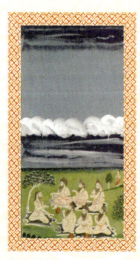

Rishi Durvasa cursing Kumbha

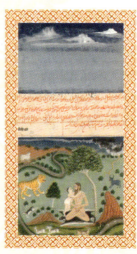

Rishi Durvasa cursing Kumbha

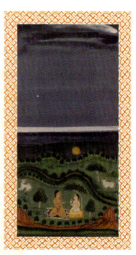

Sikhadvaja consoling Kumbha by saying that 'the thing that cannot be cured must be endured'

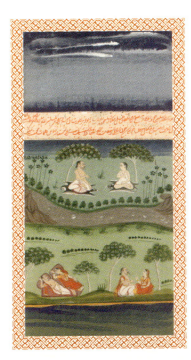 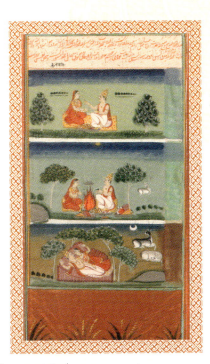

Madanika proposing to marry to follow social custom; marriage performed as per Hindu tradition before the fire; Sikhadvaja and Madanika as husband and wife

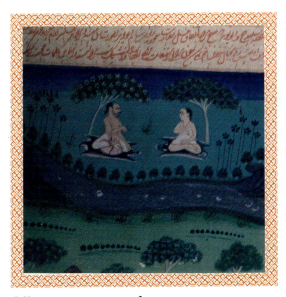

Offering prayers together

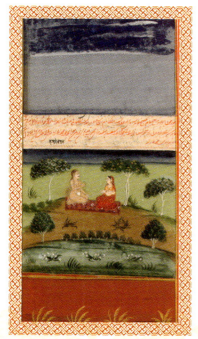

**Sikhadvaja asking: 'Who are you?
Are you Chudala?'**

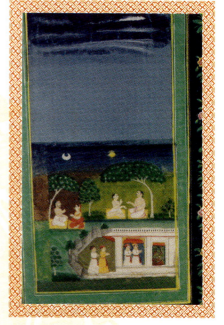

**Chudala visiting the capital to
attend to royal duties**

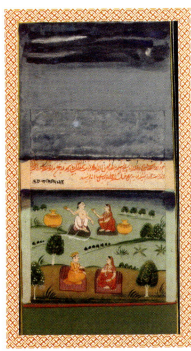

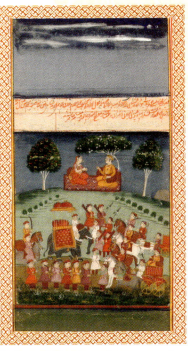

Chudala prevailing over the
king to resume his royal duties;
Raja and Rani in royal robes
after taking the sacred bath

Raja and Rani ready to mount
the royal procession

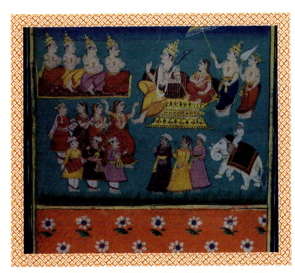

Raja Sikhadvaja and Rani Chudala ruling the
kingdom on the path of Dharma

The Story of Kaca

This story reveals that the true renunciation of all things is actually the renunciation of the ego.

Kaca the son of Brihaspati goes to his father and asks, 'Father, help me to realise my true self.' His father replies, 'Kaca, you have to renounce everything in order to be truly liberated.'

Kaca goes to the forest to renounce everything, yet he does not get peace. He again returns to his father and his father again reiterates his advice. Kaca gives up all his possessions and yet he doesn't experience inner peace.

After many years the father and son meet again; the father is saddened to learn that his son has not yet found peace. He explains to Kaca, 'Renouncing all material things but retaining your ego means you haven't realised the self. You can be truly liberated only if you affirm the divinity in yourself and renounce your ego.'

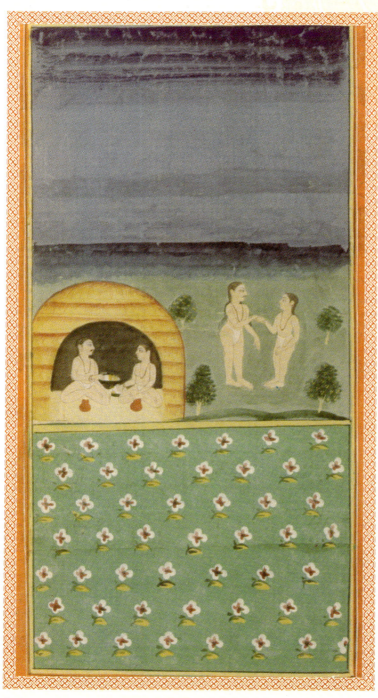

Brihaspati advising Kaca to renounce his ego and affirm the divinity in himself

The Story of Bhiringhisa

This story teaches Rama to be a great renouncer, a great doer and yet enjoy life. Bhiringhisa went to the Mahameru to meet Lord Shiva. On meeting Lord Shiva, Bhiringhisa asked his advice on how to achieve true joy. Shiva told him to be a great renouncer and a great doer and explained how this will lead him to realise the true joy of life.

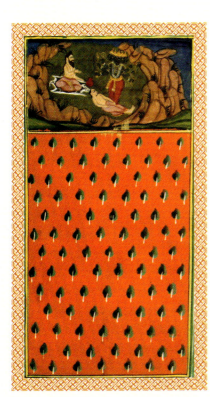

Bhiringhisa meeting Lord Shiva

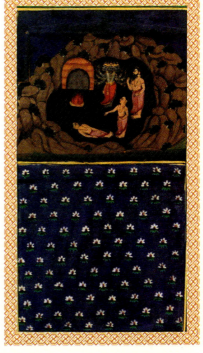

**Lord Shiva advising Bhiringhisa
to renounce the world**

The Story of Iksvaku

Through this story the philosophy of Manu is taught to Iksvaku. Iksvaku, a great king and an ancestor of Rama, begins to think that man when given worldly things has a false illusion of contentment. He is anxious to discover the truth. He goes to Manu in Bramhaloka. From Manu he learns the origin, existence and final decay of the universe – of bondage and of freedom. He also learns of the stages of self-realisation, the nature of the ego, Maya and the traits of truly liberated beings.

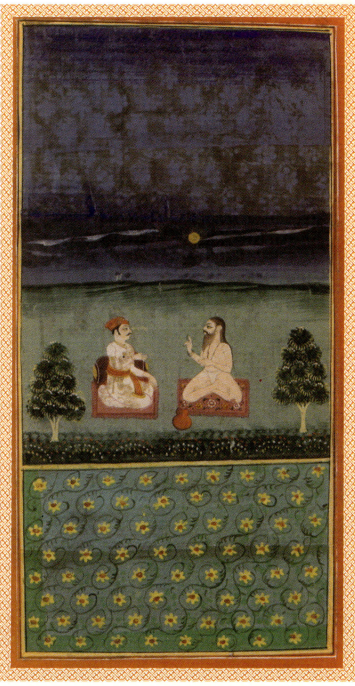

Raja Iksvaku taking lessons from Manu

The Story of a Hunter and a Sage

This story is a description of the Turiya state – a state of consciousness free from the experiences of waking, dreaming and deep-sleep.

A hunter pursues a deer which runs beyond his vision. A sage was sitting in meditation in the path the deer takes. The breathless hunter asks, 'Which way? Which way did the deer go?' The muni replies, 'I am above all states of relative experience. I do not care to know anything. Hence, I do not care which way the deer went.'

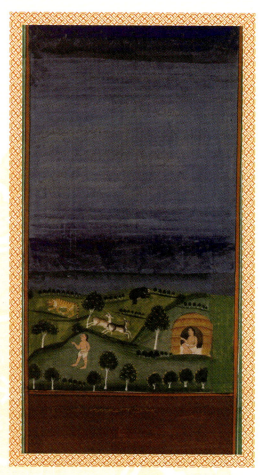

A sage free of all external forces

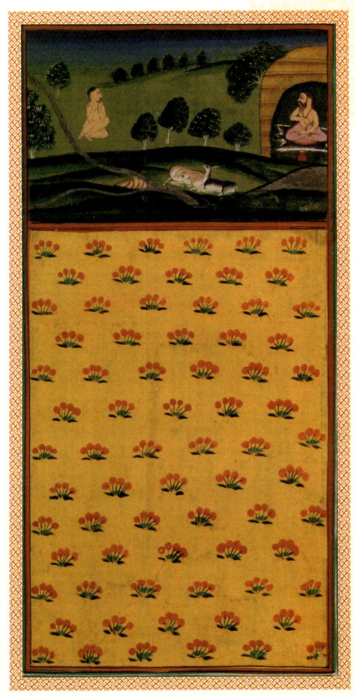

Hunter following a running deer, asking the sage about the stag

The Story of Vidya-Dhara

This story explains that in the study of the spiritual scriptures, only those who have control over their senses can benefit from them.

Vasistha once asked Bhusunda if he knew of anyone who had lived very long but could not attain self-knowledge. Bhusunda told Vasistha that there was one Vidya-Dhara who had lived for four kalpas but could not realise the self. Vidya-Dhara confessed that his passions and senses were a stumbling block in his acquiring of self-knowledge. Bhusunda taught him how to control his passions and senses and only then Vidya-dhara could realise the self.

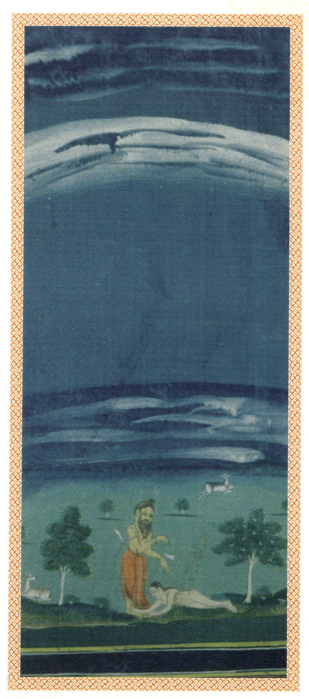

Vidya-Dhara confessing to Vasistha

The Story of Manki

This story illustrates how it is possible for a person to reach self-realisation through the teachings of another, provided his mind is prepared to imbibe the teachings.

Vasistha once came to officiate as priest in a ceremony performed by Aja. On the way he meets a bramhana called Manki. The traveller requests him to teach him how to control worldly suffering. Vasistha teaches him to overcome: 1) Savedan 2) Bhava 3) Vasana and 4) Kalana. The Brahmana practises the way to overcome the four causes of suffering and is consequently liberated.

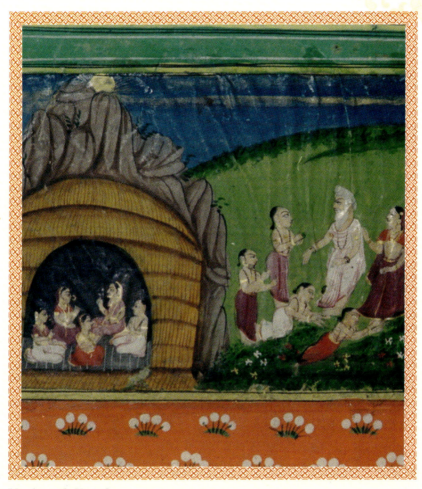

Manki with Vasistha

The Story of the Mind

This mind is like a running deer. It runs here and there in the barren land until it finds a shady tree under which to rest. For the mind the shady tree is Samadhi.

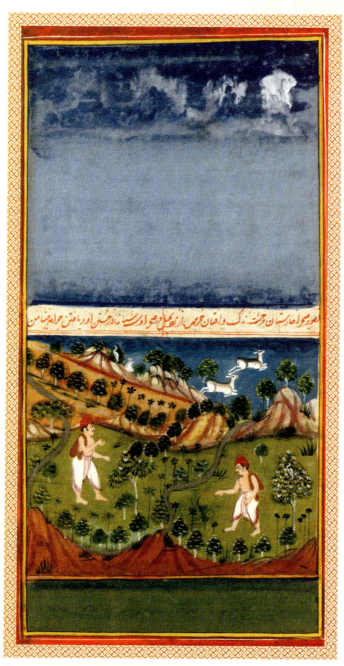

Comparison of the mind with a running deer

The Story of Vipascit

This story is among the most interesting in the *Yoga Vasistha*. This story explains how one's transmigratory carrier can be affected by one's creative power and desire.

A king named Vipascit lived in Tatamiti in the Jambu-Dvipa. Once he was attacked by enemies from all directions. He wanted to multiply himself to cope with the invasions from all four directions. To achieve this, he sacrifices his own flesh in the sacrificial fire and becomes four different Vipascits. Each Vipascit sets up a fight with an enemy and sets out in a different direction to conquer the enemy. They set out in the north, south, east and west to conquer the world. They go far and wide to different countries, die there and experience a series of transmigrations. One of them transmigrates into a deer in the zoological museum of King Dasaratha during the time Vasistha is having discourses with Rama. On hearing of the deer, Rama asks that the deer be brought to the assembly. To establish the truth, Vasistha by the power of thought changes the deer into a man and calls him Bhasa. Bhasa then recounts all his experiences to the assembly.

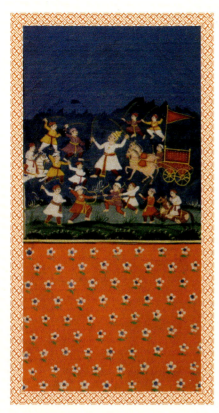

Raja Vipascit under attack by enemies

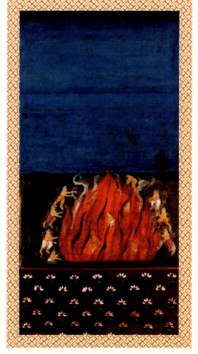

Sacrifice of Vipascit in fire

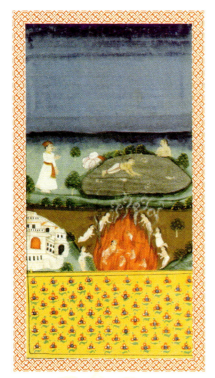

**Vipascit experiencing
transmigrations**

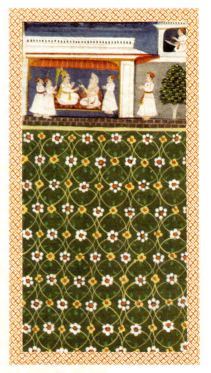

**Vasistha changing the deer into
Bhasa(man); Bhasa recounting
his experiences before Dasaratha**

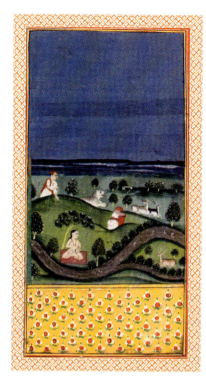

Vipascit as a deer lands in the zoo of Dasaratha

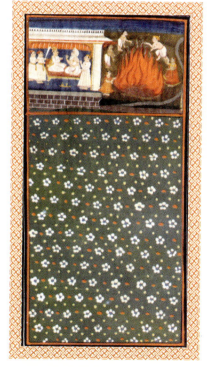

Vasistha relating the episode to Dasaratha

The Story of Sata-Rudra

The power of thought is explained through this story. It also illustrates that desires and imagination on transmigrations co-exist in the mind.

There lived a beggar, who thought of having his own house. In his dream he possesses one. Next he dreams to be a Brahaman. In this way he goes on changing his personality in hundred different forms till he becomes Rudra. Being Rudra, he is knowledgeable, living in all the hundred forms so far imagined in different worlds.

When he wakes up from the dream the imagined forms remain as distinct entities in his mind.

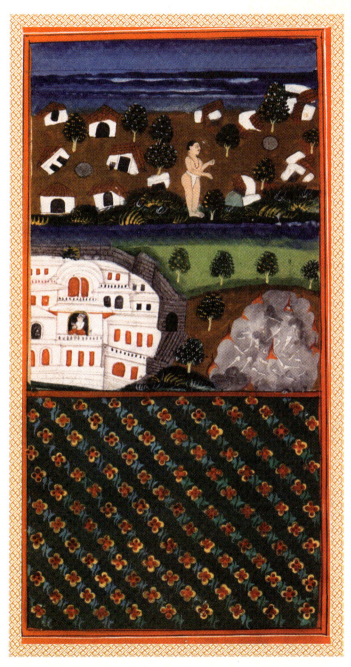

Mendicant possessing a house; imagining and living in separate worlds; mendicant by power of thought turns into Rudra

The Story of Indra

This story illustrates the possibility of the existence of the entire world within an atom.

Indra, the king of the gods, was defeated by the demons in the war. For his survival, he reduces himself and enters a sun's ray. There in imagination he rules over the world. After his death his descendants ruled there.

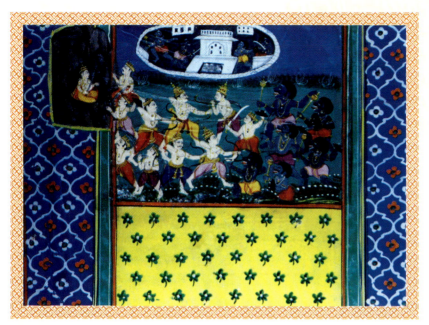

Indra, king of gods, after defeat

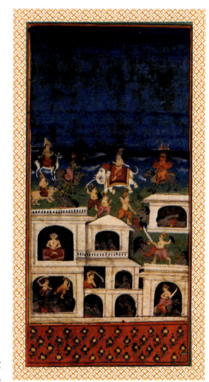

**Indra, king of gods, fighting
with demons**

The Story of a Block of Stone

The Brahman is compared to a huge rock of granite to explain that a piece of granite contains within it all the statues that can possibly be chiseled out of it. Thus, in the Brahman all the forms of the universe exist.

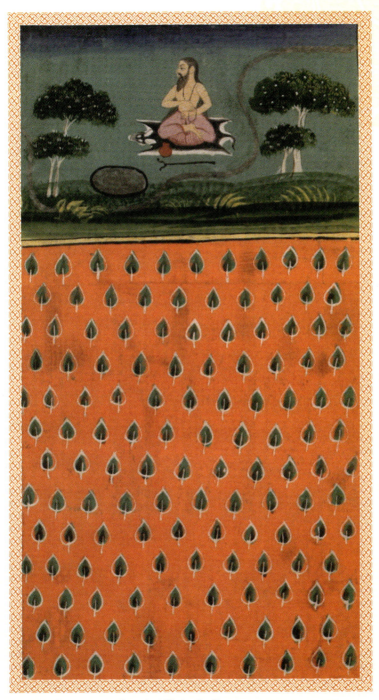

The Brahman manifest in all, including stone

CONCLUSION

Rama profusely thanked Guru Vasistha and said: 'I bow down to you my Guru; you are indeed incarnate of knowledge totally merged in the divine bliss; you are beyond duality and see only one and only one in unity of infinite.'

Rama concluded by saying, 'Sir, having received your affectionate teachings, now I am free from darkness. I shall discharge my duties as outlined by you. I have no doubts left and I am recollecting your words with full delight. I feel happier.'

Vasistha replied, 'O great Rama, it is the right time that you arise and rejoice the affectionate feelings of your people by discharging your duties towards them and live with happiness and peace.'

Vishwamitra remarked, 'O highly respected Vasistha, you have demonstrated that how great, affectionate and effective Guru you are.'

Valmiki concluded and said to Bharadvaja, 'I narrated to you the Maharamayana of the Sage Vasistha, the book on Nirvana, the ultimate objective of every person to achieve, extinction of living self.'

The learned yogis and saints in the assembly attending the discourse proclaimed, 'Rama we thank you for seeking Bramhajnana, and wish you all success and happiness to rule as an ideal king.'

The gods from the heaven applauded and felicitated Rama.

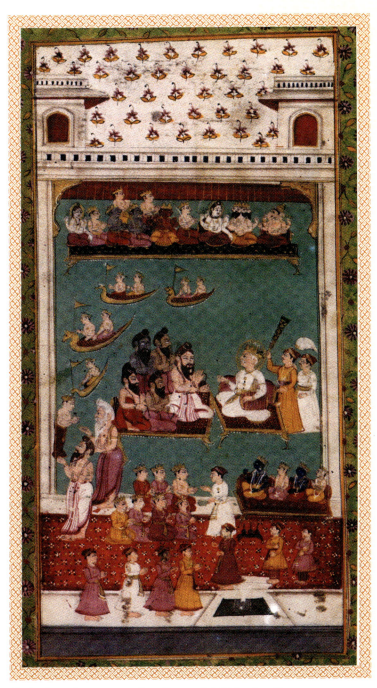

Gods from heaven applauding and felicitating Rama

INDEX OF PAINTINGS

CHAPTER IV
Upasama Prakaran

CHAPTER V
Stithi Prakaran

CHAPTER VI
Nirvana Prakaran